Sources and Traditions of Classification in Psychiatry

Sources and Traditions of Classification in Psychiatry

Edited by

Norman Sartorius
Director, Division of Mental Health, WHO

Assen Jablensky
President, Medical Academy, Sofia

Darrel A. Regier
Director, Division of Clinical Research, NIMH

Jack Denning Burke, Jr.
Director, Division of Biometry and Applied Sciences, NIMH

Robert M. A. Hirschfeld
Chief, Affective and Anxiety Disorders Research Branch,
Division of Clinical Research, NIMH

Published on behalf of the World Health Organization by

Hogrefe & Huber Publishers

Toronto • Lewiston, NY • Bern • Göttingen • Stuttgart

Library of Congress Cataloging-in-Publication Data

Sources and traditions of classification in psychiatry / Norman Sartorius ... [et al.] (editors).
p. cm.
Includes bibliographical references

1. Mental illness—Classification—History. 2. Psychiatry—Classification—History
I. Sartorius, N.
[DNLM: 1. Ethnopsychology. 2. Mental Disorders—classification. 3. Mental
Disorders—diagnosis. WM 15 S724]
RC455.2.C4S68   1990   616.89′0012—dc20   89-24610 CIP

Canadian Cataloguing in Publication Data

Main entry under title:
Sources and traditions of classification in psychiatry
Includes bibliographical references.

1. Psychology, Pathological—Diagnosis. 2. Psychology, Pathological—Classification.
3. Psychology, Pathological—History. I. Sartorius, N.
RC344.S69   1990   616.8′0475   C89-090406-5

© Copyright 1990 by WHO and Hans Huber Publishers

P. O. Box 51
Lewiston, NY 14092

12–14 Bruce Park Ave.
Toronto, Ontario M4P 2S3

ISBN 0-920887-74-0
Hans Huber Publishers • Toronto • Lewiston, NY • Bern • Stuttgart
ISBN 3-456-81821-1
Hans Huber Publishers • Bern • Stuttgart • Toronto • Lewiston, NY

Printed in Germany on acid-free paper

Preface

With regard to psychiatric classification and nomenclature all mental health workers should be bilingual: They should command both an international terminology and their own national or local professional language.

The latter is necessary for the description of phenomena relevant to psychiatric work in the specific culture, which may influence diseases and create conditions seen nowhere else. In addition, the local language may comprise words that can describe some psychiatric states with greater precision than can be obtained by means of words contained in other languages. Psychiatry is a field of considerable difficulty, and speaking about psychiatric problems demands delicate use of all resources of the language one knows best. Yet, to convey one's findings to others, an international professional language is necessary for psychiatry as well as for all other medical disciplines. Unfortunately, it is the fate of such international terminologies and classifications that they become subjects of criticism and cause severe dissatisfaction. Nobody can identify fully with them; concepts that seem necessary for many are lacking, and unfamiliar terms are introduced. These new concepts also cause anger: Why should *that* school be allowed to have some of its favorite concepts accepted, while some of *our* most useful terms are refused admittance?

In this situation the best remedy is to improve understanding of the conceptual worlds of other psychiatric schools and of the historical origin of their concepts and terms. The present volume provides the bases for such understanding. As well, the historical accounts given offer exciting reading.

Thus, for instance, the extremely complex origin of the Spanish culture in general and Spanish medicine in particular, has made it natural for J. J. López-Ibor to follow the roots of Spanish psychiatry—Arab, Greek, Roman—back to antiquity. In contrast, A. V. Snezhnevsky shows how a new classification and terminology of the major psychoses has developed within Russian psychiatry during a few decades, based on detailed studies of course and symptomatology.

For non-Francophone psychiatrists who have looked upon French psychiatry with great respect but a minimum of understanding, P. Pichot's chapter will be much welcomed for help. German psychiatry has had great impact on all other psychiatric schools, especially through its description of the endogenous psychoses: J. Glatzel's account shows how much German psychiatry has contributed in many other directions.

An overview of psychiatric literature during the 1980s might give the impression that American psychiatric thinking is mainly concentrated on DSM-III. G. Klerman's chapter gives abundant evidence to the contrary, showing how versatile American psychiatry has been over the years—and still is.

R. E. Kendell's account of English psychiatry illustrates, among other things, the great importance British research has had for the establishment for a solid foundation of international classifications.

In P. Bech's chapter, an account is given of the important position the psychogenic (reactive) psychoses have held in the Scandinavian countries since the beginning of this century.

N. Wig provides overwhelming evidence for the importance of including concepts which are indispensable for work in developing countries into any international classification.

The rich and interesting material presented in this volume will undoubtedly lead to more benevolent, understanding attitudes toward the difficult attempts at creating international psychiatric classifications. This is of particular importance now that the 10th Revision of the International Classification of Diseases is about to enter into worldwide long-lasting use.

Erik Strömgren

Table of Contents

Table of Contents

Editors' Foreword

In the early 1960s, the World Health Organization initiated a major international program in order to stimulate research leading to an improvement of psychiatric diagnosis and to standardize strategies about mental disorders. The program brought together experts in psychiatry and public health specialists from some 30 countries and produced several important results over the years. It has facilitated the dialogue among representatives of psychiatric schools, and between them and public health specialists. It has developed, adapted or tested in an international setting joint ratings of videotaped interviews and other methods for the study of diagnosis in psychiatry. It has produced numerous proposals for the improvement of the classification of mental disorders, among which was the inclusion of a glossary describing the content of each of the categories grouping mental disorders into the 8th Revision of the International Classification of Diseases. A network of individuals and centers working on matters concerned with psychiatric disease classification was established [1, 2] and continued its existence.

The next decade saw continuing growth of interest in psychiatric classification, perhaps in part stimulated by WHO's efforts, but certainly fueled by the burgeoning of research on new methods of treatment and by the growing number of contacts between psychiatrists worldwide. International travel became easier, psychiatric conferences mushroomed, and several international collaborative studies opened the doors to other worlds of psychiatry even further. Several national classifications accompanied by criteria of varying precision were produced, aiming to facilitate understanding among scientists. Among these the efforts of the American Psychiatric Association embodied in the DSM III did the most to bring about a general acceptance of the need for agreed (operational) criteria and a comprehensive classification that can be used for various tasks within psychiatry.

In the late 1970s, the World Health Organization, in collaboration with the US Alcohol, Drug Abuse and Mental Health Administration, established an international program on classification and diagnosis of mental disorders, alcohol and drug-related problems [3]. This program started with a series of workshops in which groups of scientists representing different psychiatric traditions and cultures met to review available knowledge and identify areas for future research. The findings and recommendations of the working groups were reviewed in a major international conference [4], resulting in material and guidelines for future work.

Several of the recommendations of the conference led to major research projects. A project involving centers in 17 countries was started to develop an instrument suitable for epidemiological studies of mental disorders in different countries [5]. Another collaborative study was launched to develop an instrument for the assessment of the mental state by clinicians [6]; and yet another also involving centers in many countries to develop an internationally applicable personality disorder examination [7]. A series of Lexicons systematically providing definitions for terms used in the 9th and 10th Revisions of the International Classification of Diseases, as well as numerous other terms, is being published [8]. While these projects were getting underway, the task of producing definitions of criteria for use in conjunction with the 10th revision of the ICD became imminent. The synchrony of work on instruments and on criteria for the ICD proved to be beneficial: The development of instruments helped in operationalizing criteria for the ICD and vice versa—the discussions about the classification found their reflections in the shape and content of the assessment instruments.

Another one of the recommendations of the Copenhagen conference was that the views of different psychiatric schools should be presented in a (single) volume to facilitate the understanding of origins of the classification proposed for international use from 1990 onwards. It was with this goal in mind that the Steering Committee of the joint WHO/ADAMHA project has assembled the views of most major psychiatric schools (or groups of schools) and presents them in this publication to the world's scientific community. The papers brought together in this volume have been prepared by leading authorities thoroughly conversant with their respective subject. As a result, the various chapters present a panorama of psychiatric thinking over time in different sociocultural settings. The papers highlight the origins of concepts, some of which have gained wide currency in contemporary psychiatry, while others have given rise to critical debate. They demonstrate both similarities in approach or philosophy and still existent differences. A number of them are already bridged in practice, and others can probably be overcome, too. But there is little hope that progress toward creating a language all concerned can understand will be made until all those involved listen very carefully to what the others are saying. It is the editors' hope that this book should make it easier to do so.

There is no doubt about the need to continue work that will eventually lead to diagnostic criteria linked to internationally applicable and acceptable instruments for psychiatric assessment and to standardized and largely automated information systems which will make it possible to plan, evaluate and steer psychiatric services or carry out epidemiological, biological and other research on mental illness.

Once this effort of description and processing of information is further advanced, it is likely that differences between psychiatric schools will become less noticeable and less easy to maintain. This will not make the descriptions of views of the schools presented here epistemologically and historically less valuable. On the contrary, they will gain in importance because they will continue to remind us that much that was achieved could only be reached because of the contributions, over the years, of many people and in many lands of this one world.

References

1) Kramer, M., Sartorius, N., Jablensky, A., Gulbinat, W. The ICD-9 classification of mental disorders: A review of its development and contents. *Acta psych. scand.* (1979) 59, 241–262

2) Sartorius, N. Classification: An international perspective. *Psychiatric Annals* 6: 8 August 1976

3) Jablensky, A., Sartorius, N., Hirschfeld, R. and Pardes, H. Diagnosis and classification of mental disorders and alcohol- and drug-related problems: A research agenda for the 1980s. *Psychological Medicine* (1983) 13, 907–921)

4) *Mental disorders, alcohol- and drug-related problems—International perspectives on their diagnosis and classification.* Reports and recommendations of the International Conference on Diagnosis and Classification of Mental Disorders and Alcohol- and Drug-Related Problems, Copenhagen, April 1982. Excerpta Medica 1985.

5) Robins, L., Wing, J., Wittchen, H.-U., Helzer, J. E., Babor, T. F., Burke, J., Farmer, A., Jablensky, A., Pickens, R., Regier, D. A., Sartorius, N. and Towle, L. E. The Composite International Diagnostic Interview. *Arch. Gen. Psychiatry* (1988) 45, 1069–1077

6) Wing, J. K., Babor, T., Brugha, T., Burke, J., Cooper, J. E., Giel, R., Jablensky, A., Regier, D. and Sartorius, N. SCAN: Schedules for Clinical Assessment in Neuropsychiatry. *Arch. Gen. Psychiatry* (in press)

7) Loranger, A. W., Hirschfeld, R. M. A., Sartorius, N. and Regier, D. A. *The International Personality Disorder Examination: A semistructured clinical interview for use with DSM-III-R and ICD-10 in different cultures.* In press

8) *Lexicon of psychiatric and mental health terms, Volume 1.* WHO (1989).

1
Sources and Traditions of Psychiatric Classification: Introduction

Norman Sartorius*

A classification is a way of seeing the world. It is the reification of an ideological position, of an accepted standard of theory and knowledge. Classifying means creating, defining or confirming boundaries of concepts. Through these, in turn, we define ourselves, our future and our past, the territory of our discipline, its importance and its exclusiveness. No other intellectual act is of such importance: If our classifications of things and people in the world around us were to collapse, the world would cease to exist as a coherent and organized whole and would become a nebulous agglomeration of rubbish—matter, people and things out of place.

Classifications of diseases in psychiatry were at the center of interest not only among psychiatrists but also among lawyers, philosophers, taxonomists and many others even before psychiatry as a medical discipline came into existence. In part this arose because the absence of physical signs and laboratory abnormalities in many psychiatric disorders makes psychiatric disorders much more dependent on the consensus of what in a given society is normal, what is abnormal, what is asocial and what is part of a disease. In part, also, the interest in psychiatric classification springs from the intermingling of understandable and incomprehensible behavior, from the frequency of psychiatric symptoms in the normal population and from the absence of specific treatments that would allow a classification *ex juvantibus*. Many of the conditions that could be the subjects of psychiatric classification are of unknown origin, have a variable course and an uncertain outcome; epistemologically, they have a low rank and present formidable difficulties for placement into a classification of diseases. In the absence of convincing evidence, some continue to consider psychiatric disorders to be similar to ailments in general medicine and thus eventually

---

* Director, Division of Mental Health, World Health Organization, Geneva, Switzerland. Some of the arguments presented here have been included in the article "International Perspectives of Psychiatric Classification" by the author, published in *The British Journal of Psychiatry*, 152 (May 1988), pp. 9–14.

definable as diseases, with specific causes, symptoms, course and outcome; others—with just as much conviction—preach the view that
psychiatric problems are responses that are not specific to causes and
therefore not appropriate to a system that classifies disease entities.

In spite of its promise, so prominent in the 1960s, research during the
past two decades failed to provide evidence that could help to create
disease concepts and disease entities in psychiatry. Syndromes—such
as schizophrenia or depression—are still widely used, and most attempts to create coherent links between clinical symptoms, specific
causal factors, pathogenetic models and prognostic types have failed.
The numerous findings that the neurosciences, relying on apparatus of
ever-increasing sophistication, have produced about the functioning of
the brain have not been accompanied by any significant advance in the
understanding of ways in which structures or processes in the brain are
translated into mental functioning, or on how brain relates to mind. In
part this was because new methods of investigation appeared so
rapidly that there was a delay in the accumulation of data necessary to
define limits of normality for the findings of such investigation; in part,
however, this was also because of the growing distance between the
neuroscientists, clinicians and epistemologists.

Some of the previously held views also form an obstacle to agreement on a classification or to improving it. The continuing insistence,
for example, on the mind-body dichotomy inherent in some of the
classification systems which emerged in the 19th century is such a
constraint. Discontinuous with earlier European views and at odds
with philosophies of other cultures, this dichotomy was an expression
of the reductionist tendencies of the industrial revolution and, at the
time, was useful in furthering the understanding of diseases and research. Today, however, this is not so: Other ways of thinking about
health and disease, mind and body, mental and physical, individual
and social are needed if we are to formulate creative hypotheses and
design investigations likely to result in breakthroughs in our knowledge about mental illness.

Furthermore, recent years brought with them a significant increase
in the recognition of cultural constraints to agreement on diagnostic
and classificatory systems. Most of these are well known and do not
need enumeration. Some, however, are less obvious and therefore more
difficult to tackle. Such, for example, is the difference between the ways
in which time is conceptualized and used in the description of phenomena; such is also the difference between cultures in their tolerance for
unresolved conflict and contradiction. Those who can or even prefer to
maintain indeterminacy do not accept working with classifications requiring immediate final assignment to classes on the basis of incomplete information.

The improvement of communication with psychiatrists from Third World countries and an increase in respect for what they have to say has, among other results, brought out the unresolved issues in psychiatric classifications in the industrialized countries. One of those, for example, is the issue of classification of acute psychoses—the frequent, undifferentiated conditions with reasonably good prognosis which make up a large proportion of all emergency admissions to psychiatric facilities and which seem almost to fit descriptions of a variety of conditions, such as psychogenic psychoses, cycloid psychoses and reactive psychoses. Another issue is the classification of conditions with somatic presentation usually bypassing psychiatric services. Yet a further one is the personality disorders whose degree of abnormality is very dependent on prevailing sociocultural norms and on our views about the likelihood that personality traits can be changed in time or by intervention.

The organization of helping agencies and arrangements for care have in recent years led to a decrease in agreement on classification. The growing diversity of services, for example, and the increasing separation between systems that administer them led to the development of different "service languages." General health care personnel now deal with many mentally ill people and develop classifications they find easy to use. The growing complexity of health insurance accounting has led to a language and classification that is used and useful within that system, but that can be only partially linked to classifications used in health services. Classifications and language conventions for a variety of other purposes and for different social service sectors have mushroomed in many countries and serve well in practice. Unfortunately, the mushrooming of jargons and classification schemes has not been paralleled by efforts to ensure that they can be translated into a reference classification. As a result, in many settings the same condition changes labels as patients pass through health care, research and social welfare facilities, and any attempt to pool information from different systems becomes an expensive utopia. At the same time, the development of long-term care in a complex health and social service system has brought with it the need to produce classifications reflecting adequately the many characteristics and requirements of the individual entering the system. Multi-axial classification schemes have made a major contribution in this respect; but even where they are applied, significant unanswered public health and practical needs remain. The number of patients, for example, who have several impairments and diseases—all encodable on the same axis and all relevant to care and outcome—is constantly increasing because of longer life expectancy in general, better chances of survival and improved diagnostic possibilities; ways of classifying the multitude of problems in an individual, particularly when these require interventions by different social sectors or medical disciplines, have not yet been developed.

Developments that have little to do with the changes in our understanding of psychiatric disorders have also had an impact on the classificatory scene. The support of the pharmaceutical industry for work on classification and the impact of requirements of drug regulatory agencies requesting investigators to specify the diagnostic system used in drug trials led to a striking increase of interest in psychiatric classification. On the other hand, recent difficulties in the use of psychiatric registers, resulting *inter alia* from the upsurge of interest in the rights of the mentally ill and the significant decentralization of data collection (for example, to the federal, state or even county level), decreased possibilities that data could be pooled; and the starvation budgets given to public health agencies in many industrial countries led to a sharp decrease of interest in work on classifications among public-health-oriented psychiatrists. Paradoxically, the leadership in classification research has thus shifted from psychiatrists with a main interest in public health to those engaged in treatment research.

In many countries, national societies have undertaken and completed revisions of their classification. The most spectacular of these is the classification proposed by the American Psychiatric Association (DSM-III, the DSM-III-R and the Research Diagnostic Criteria); but important developments have also appeared in many other settings ranging from the publication of the elaborate glossary of psychiatric syndromes for epidemiological research in the USSR to the child mental disorder classification and the operational criteria for psychosis in French-speaking countries and the Indonesian classification and glossary. While immensely interesting and advancing our knowledge, this upsurge in the creation of national classificatory systems is also puzzling: It is difficult to understand reasons for its occurrence.

Kraepelin's classification was not the only one in Germany at the time; it represented the views of a professional offered to his pupils and fellows in the country and elsewhere—as a hypothesis open for everyone's use. Nationalist feelings in the allegiance of psychiatric schools have the appearance of nationalist feelings in the political sphere some 100 years ago: The need for national identification has appeared at an unexpectedly late moment in the history of classification, research and practice. Financial gain that can be obtained by producing and copyrighting a classification only partially explains this development. The unprecedented rivalry between professions each feeling that it will be legitimized once it has its own classification of diseases may also be invoked in seeking causes for it.

These and other developments threatened to obliterate gains made in the 1960s in understanding among scientists, clinicians and decision makers. This would have been a pity at any time, but in the early 1990s it is a major menace to further progress of scientific discovery and improvement of care worldwide. Technology of communication and computing now makes it possible to pool vast quantities of data and thus detect trends and regularities that have not been accessible to discovery or analysis ever before. Without a common language these technological advances cannot be employed. The heightened priority and visibility of mental health services requires an efficient system of monitoring its function; for without a common usage and understanding of terms such an evaluation is meaningless. The rapid development of treatment techniques requires their continuous assessment which is unthinkable without an agreement on diagnosis and assessment of change.

These considerations were among the reasons for launching a major project on diagnosis and classification in 1980. This international effort, sponsored jointly by WHO and ADAMHA, started with an intensive review of the present state of diagnosis and classification, identifying gaps in knowledge and defining priorities and methodological requirements for multicenter research to overcome them. It continued by the implementation of several major international studies, aiming to produce assessment instruments that will be applicable in different cultures, glossaries, classification proposals, and reviews of knowledge relevant to diagnosis and classification.

A number of results from this project are already available. Networks of centers in some 30 countries, for example, collaborate in the testing of several instruments suitable for cross-cultural application and allow a comprehensive and reliable assessment of the mental state of patients in different countries. Lexical descriptions for psychiatric terms have been developed on the basis of contributions from experts from around the world. Numerous consultations with creators of national psychiatric classifications seem to offer hope that these classificatory systems will be translatable into an international reference classification.

The experience obtained in the project so far is rich and allows more rational priority setting in research on diagnosis and classification. It also allows—combined with results of trials of the 10th Revision of the International Classification of Diseases currently in process in 195 centers in 55 countries—to define principles that should govern the shape and content of a classification offered for universal use. Such a system should:

1) be based on points of agreement among mental health professionals, and between them and other users of the classification;

2) be sufficiently simple and understandable to allow easy use by those who will deal with commonly encountered disorders;

3) at all times be a servant rather than a master of classifications in existence. It must not aim to oust, compete with or replace regional or local classifications, which often have valuable functions and are likely to be well adjusted to the situation in which they have come into existence;

4) be sufficiently well liked as a tool of information exchange to generate translations of national or special-purpose classifications into the reference classification;

5) be rather conservative and theoretically unenterprising so as to remain attractive or at least acceptable to a wide variety of people of different orientations and knowledge;

6) be stable and abide by the rule that changes can only be introduced when sufficient scientific data have become available to support the change and facilitate its acceptance;

7) take into account languages into or from which the classification will be translated;

8) preserve a certain amount of continuity between successive revisions, for economic and scientific reasons.

The development of a classification corresponding to these requirements is not an easy task; its realization requires numerous scientific health-political and organizational steps. An essential requirement, however, in this process—common to all the necessary steps—is to examine the positions and promises inherent in currently used classifications with respect and with a determination to use the best of available knowledge, regardless of its source.

2

The Diagnosis and Classification of Mental Disorders in the French-Speaking Countries: Background, Current Values and Comparison with other Classifications

P. Pichot*

This chapter deals with French psychiatric diagnosis and classification as it differs from other standard national or international concepts and terminology. Attention focuses on two popular French diagnostic categories: the two groups of disorders known in France as transitory delusional states (bouffées délirantes) and chronic delusional states.**

Because these two uniquely French nosological concepts overlap with several standard psychiatric entities there can be no one-to-one correspondence between French and other recognized nomenclatures, although, as will be shown, almost identical diagnostic criteria for some of the conditions they circumscribe are found in the latest classifications, such as the most recent edition of the World Health Organization's *International Classification of Diseases* (ICD-9) and the 1980 edition of the American Psychiatric Association's *Diagnostic and Statistical Manual of Mental Disorders* (DSM-III).

Background

Understanding the distinctive features of French psychiatric thought requires some familiarity with developments in both German and

* 24 rue des Fossés Saint Jacques, 75005 Paris, France.
** Mental instability (déséquilibre mental), although a specifically French diagnostic concept, shares almost identical criteria with ICD-9 301.7, "Personality disorder with predominantly sociopathic or asocial manifestation." As a concept it played an interesting role in the history of French psychiatry—which, however, is beyond the scope of this chapter.

French psychiatry between 1880 and World War I. By 1880, France could look back on a century of leadership in the field of psychiatry. The achievements of early French exponents such as Philippe Pinel, Jean Etienne Esquirol and others were widely respected abroad. When, in 1851, J. P. Falret described a "new species" of mental disorder consisting of periodic mood swings (later to be known as manic-depressive illness, circular type [DSM-III] and subsequently bipolar disorder [DSM-III]), his courteous but unyielding academic debate before the Imperial Academy of Medicine over the primacy of discovery was followed overseas with as much official attention as in France.*

The persecutory delusions originally described in 1852 by Charles Lasègue—and in 1878 by Jean Pierre Falret—are of particular relevance to this chapter. The same holds true for Benedict Morel's description in 1853 of a type of psychosis observed in young people, for which he coined the term démence précoce, the exact model in French of dementia praecox, its Latin translation.

In 1857, Morel also published his *Treatise on the Degeneracies*, which introduced terrain or hereditary constitution as a principle of classification. Until the eve of World War I, Morel's theory of degeneracy was widely used both in France and abroad** as a framework for interpreting clinical observation; it was to become the cornerstone of French psychiatry just a few decades after its publication.

Psychiatry had begun to come into its own in the German-speaking world around 1800, and Emil Kraepelin was the first German psychiatrist to make a significant mark on international psychiatric nomenclature. In the successive editions of his *Textbook of Psychiatry* Kraepelin gradually evolved a system of classification to which all subsequent systems have paid tribute. In the fifth edition (1896) he notes that he has "(taken) the final, decisive step (leading) from the symptomatic to the clinical viewpoint . . . (because it has become clear in all areas that) causes, clinical course and outcome better define specific mental disorders than loose collections of symptoms."***

In describing those conditions known today as functional psychoses, Kraepelin leaned more heavily on the diagnostic axes of clinical course

---

* A full account of the presentation and rebuttal appeared in the *American Journal of Insanity*.

** Between 1908 and 1915, for instance, 28 articles on or relating in one way or another to degeneracy appeared in the *American Journal of Insanity*.

*** . . . den letzten, entscheidenden Schritt von der symptomatischen zur klinischen Betrachtungsweise . . ., (da) überall hat die Bedeutung der äußeren Krankheitszeichen hinter den Gesichtspunkten zurücktreten müssen, die sich aus den Entstehungsbedingungen, aus Verlauf und Ausgang der einzelnen Störungen ergeben haben.

and prognosis than on etiology, which he discussed only superficially and hypothetically. He distinguished three classes of psychoses: manic-depressive psychoses, dementia praecox (a generic term for hebephrenia, catatonia and paranoid dementia) and paranoia. While Kraepelin was perfecting his nomenclature in Germany, French psychiatric thinking stood under the compelling sway of Valentin Magnan, the man and his theories. Magnan used a modified version of Morel's theory of degeneracy as the backbone of his own classification system. He separated the functional psychoses into two categories, each of which he believed to be directly correlated with the type of hereditary constitutions on which they occurred. He thought that individuals of sound stock were constitutionally "predisposed" to develop particular types of mental disorders, and degenerates others. He believed the disorders we know today as affective psychoses occurred only among the predisposed normal population. The remaining functional psychoses he divided into two classes: chronic delusional state of systematic evolution* which, he believed, occurred, like the affective psychoses, only in the predisposed (normal) population, and delusional states of degeneracy which he thought could occur, as the term suggests, only in degenerates.

Chronic delusional state of systematic evolution is the pivot of Magnan's classification. Indeed, delusional states of degeneracy constitute a miscellaneous assortment of all non-affective functional psychoses that deviate in any significant way from the tidy clinical picture of the chronic delusional state, based on Lasègue's and Falret's delusions of persecution and described by Magnan in the following terms:

Chronic delusional state usually occurs in adults who have never previously shown signs of disordered mind, manner or mood. The main characteristics are protracted course (up to 50 years or more) and relentlessly invariable progression through four easily recognizable consecutive phases, with distinctively contrasting affective tone in the second and third phases.

The first or prodromal phase is characterized by illusions, miscalculations, faulty judgement and growing fretfulness. The second or persecutory phase consists of excruciating, mostly auditory, hallucinations, signs of neurological malfunctioning and delusions of persecution. The third, or grandiose phase, is recognized by fanciful hallucinations, signs of neurological malfunctioning and grandiosity. In the fourth or terminal phase, understanding decays: this is the

---

* This is a rather literal and ponderous translation of the French délire chronique à évolution systématique, Magnan's original term. It has been left in this somewhat awkward form in English in deference to the original translation by A. Marie and J. MacPherson of the twelve lectures by Doctor Magnan on the subject, published in English in the *American Journal of Insanity* (1895–1896). The only concession to modern usage made here has been to substitute the euphemism "delusional states" for the now contaminated term "insanity," which appeared in Marie and MacPherson's original version.

period of dementia. These four consecutive phases consistently follow the same inalterable sequence.

All delusional states departing from this sharply defined pattern were relegated to the catchall delusional states of degeneracy. In other words, any significant deviation from the standard clinical course was taken as proof of underlying degeneracy.

Depending on their native endowment, degenerates were considered to fall into two distinct groups: (1) *inferior degenerates*, a group embracing idiots, imbeciles and morons, and (2) *superior degenerates* exhibiting such "stigmata of degeneracy" as aberrant psychological and emotional traits and "even obsessions or compulsions"—in other words, manifestations of what we would today call personality disorders. In some instances the stigmata of the underlying degenerate personality were measured only by the degree of observable deviation from the standard diagnostic pattern for chronic delusional state of systematic evolution.

In Magnan's classification, the delusional states of degeneracy comprise three rubrics: delusional states of inferior degenerates; chronic delusional states deviating from the sharply defined clinical course of chronic delusional state of systematic evolution, e.g., those commencing with delusions of grandeur; and acute delusional states called transitory delusional states of degeneracy, a concept on which we now focus our attention.

Transitory Delusional States

The classical description of transitory delusional states was given in 1886 by Magnan's student Legrain. Five points serve as diagnostic criteria:

1) *Sudden onset:* "Like a bolt from the blue full-blown delusions suddenly shatter the poise of a fully rational mind . . . and flare up without premonitory signs." Moreover, there is no precipitating event or at most only minimal identifiable stress. Magnan and Legrain considered sudden onset to be the main sign of a favourable short-term prognosis.

2) *Characteristics of the delusions:* The delusions are ripe from the outset. "There is no warning sign. The delusions form and lurk fully developed in the mind, then burst forth with overpowering force, but fail to evolve further." The delusional themes are numerous, diverse and protean, e.g., persecutory, grandiose, mystical, erotic, and so forth, sometimes "impossible to define." The delusions are a loose, shifting, motley jumble, disorganized, without recognizable struc-

ture or cohesiveness. They may be accompanied by a kaleidoscopic "parade" of neurological symptoms: illusions and related pathological inferences, or hallucinations of one or more of the senses of perception. Hallucinations, however, are secondary to, and not an essential feature of, the disorder; transitory delusional states may occur without concomitant hallucinations. The delusions overpower the mind and block insight. "Degenerates are completely caught up in and overwhelmed by the delusions from the outset."

3) *Clouded consciousness associated with emotional instability:* A certain degree of confusion can be demonstrated and there are symptoms ranging from anxiety, agitation, impulsiveness and expansiveness to inertia.

4) *Absence of physical signs:* The disorder is limited to psychological and emotional symptoms and does not affect physical health; vital signs and the major bodily functions remain without physiological limits throughout.

5) *Rapid remission:* Quick return to the premorbid level of functioning is an essential diagnostic criterion (the French term bouffée [= flare-up or outburst] implies suddenness of both onset and resolution). The delusions "often vanish with the same rapidity with which they have cropped up," in a few hours, days or weeks. "By definition, transitory delusional states are short-lived." Nevertheless, because of the unstable underlying degenerative constitution, relapses may occur. Vulnerability to delusional states always remains. A well-known French aphorism proclaims "C'est un délire sans conséquence, sinon sans lendemain" (roughly, "Through the mind go again, no scars remain"). When recurring delusional states are "separated by symptom-free intervals," Magnan speaks of recurrent transitory delusional state (bouffée délirante à type intermittent).

Toward the end of the century, Magnan's system was dogma. Its two classes of mental disorder—chronic delusional state in the predisposed but constitutionally normal population and the delusional states of degeneracy, the most significant of which were the transitory delusional states—permeated all psychiatric thought. For 20 years Magnan's diagnostic criteria were actively referred to and applied, though subjected to continuous revisions.

Around 1910, classification based on the theory of degeneracy fell into disuse. Nevertheless, the term transitory delusional states has survived as a popular diagnosis, a relic of Morel's theory of degeneracy and a tribute to Magnan's influence.

Chronic Delusional States

The introduction of Kraepelin's nomenclature posed two stubborn problems for French psychiatrists: (1) how to reconcile Magnan's doctrine with Kraepelin's dementia praecox; (2) how to differentiate between dementia praecox and the essentially identical term démence précoce, coined earlier by Morel.

This dilemma marked the beginning of what was to be prolonged resistance to Kraepelin's principles, apparent compromise notwithstanding. In the final analysis, the unsurmountable obstacles to establishing workable one-to-one correlations with Kraepelin's system have engendered particularities in the present-day French subdivisions of chronic delusional states which are sometimes difficult to pigeonhole in other nomenclatures. The history of this struggle has been admirably outlined by B. Bonfils in his doctoral thesis (1979) *Histoire du concept de démence précoce en France* (see References, Appendix 2).

It soon became apparent that Magnan's chronic delusional state of systematic evolution was a misleading construct, defining a disorder found more readily in theory than in practice, the exception more than the rule. While French clinicians piled up description after description of chronic delusional states infringing on Kraepelin's paranoia and many cases of his paranoid form of dementia praecox, the boundaries between chronic delusional state of systematic evolution and chronic delusional states of degeneracy gradually became blurred. As a result, there evolved a new French classification which sorts out chronic delusional states, irrespective of presumptive hereditary constitution, according to predominant symptomatology viewed as the "delusional mechanism." This shift in perspective was eventually to result in the current French classification, which divides all "non-schizophrenic" chronic delusional states into three or—in the case of INSERM nomenclature—four diagnostic groups.

Chronic Interpretive Psychosis

Interpretive Delusional State

In 1909, Sérieux and Capgras described as chronic non-hallucinatory delusional states a group of disorders which they subdivided into three classes: interpretive, imaginative and vindicative delusional states. The subordinate category interpretive delusional state*, still known today

---

* In *Les folies raisonnantes. Le délire d'interprétation*, Paris, 1909. This book was reviewed by Ernest Jones under the original French title in the *American Journal of Insanity*, 66 (1909–1910), p. 182.

in the French-speaking world as the Sérieux and Capgras-type interpretive delusional state, figures prominently in current French classification. The authors define it as a "chronic, systematized psychosis feeding on delusional interpretations and developing gradually in vulnerable individuals, without conspicuous neurological impairment, not resulting in dementia despite its prolonged course." The core of the psychosis is constituted by "false reasoning originating in the misinterpretation of correctly perceived fact or facts, to which logical but erroneous inferences lend misconstrued subjective meaning consonant with personal inclinations, sentiments and preoccupations." Sérieux and Capgras list the following diagnostic criteria: (1) the complexity and coherence of the delusions; (2) the absence of hallucinations or their manifest subordination to the delusional core; (3) unimpaired intelligence; (4) progressive extension of the delusional network; (5) incurability without significant mental or social deterioration.

The interpretive delusional state of French nomenclature resembles Kraepelin's paranoia. In fact, in subsequent French usage, the terms interpretive and paranoiac have often been employed interchangeably to describe the same delusional states. However, because the French diagnostic criteria are more flexible, disorders best classified under this heading are diagnosed more frequently in France than is the paranoia vera of German authors (see Figure 2).

(Emotional)* Delusional States

Among the chronic non-hallucinatory psychoses, Sérieux and Capgras also differentiated a group of disorders they called vindicative delusional states. They described this group as "chronic, systematized psychoses, in which a single, relentless and patently pathological thought or thought complex, intensified by opposition, subdues and dominates all other mental activity." The features they ascribed to vindicative delusional states are quite similar to those of Kraepelin's *Querulanten-wahn*. Specifically French, however, is the classification of vindicative and sentimental delusional states under one rubric, (emotional) delusional states, and their ultimate differentiation from (intellectual) delu-

---

* "(Emotional)" as well as "(intellectual)," which appears later on in this text, are both contrived terms of convenience used here to underscore two broad subdivisions with the framework of chronic interpretive psychosis. While this dichotomy is in general implicitly recognized in the French literature, it is not specifically sanctioned by explicit French terminology. Brackets are used throughout this chapter to indicate the deviation from French practice. For further explanation see Footnote, Figure 1; Legend, Figure 2 and Bilingual Glossary, Appendix 1.

sional states, which include hypersensitive and interpretive delusional states per se (see Figure 2).

This differentiation was particularly well delineated around 1930 by G. de Clérambault, when he wrote his classical description of erotic paranoia. According to this author sentimental (= conjugal + erotic) delusional states are characterized, on the one hand, by a central delusional premise, a single permanent and unshakable but erroneous conviction (for instance, "I am the victim of an injustice" in the case of vindicative delusional states; "she is unfaithful to me" in conjugal paranoia; "he loves me" in erotic paranoia) and, on the other hand, by an elaboration of a particular sub-theme derived from that central delusional premise—the feature he felt distinguished them from the interpretive delusional state.

But because the "delusional mechanism" is interpretative in all instances, French psychiatrists have since usually failed to draw a fine line of demarcation between (intellectual) and (emotional) delusional states, and rather tend to view them as subordinate classes of one broad category, that is to say, of chronic interpretive psychosis or paranoia, as defined by the more elastic but well-documented criteria of French nomenclature (see Figure 2).

Chronic Hallucinatory Psychosis

In 1911, Gilbert Ballet published an article entitled "Chronic hallucinatory psychosis." He expanded his description of this clinical entity in 1913. Even though there had previously been similar reports, Ballet's paper is considered to be the first one authenticating the disorder. The diagnostic criteria are:

a) persistent hallucinatory activity: The hallucinations of this disorder were classified in the 1920s by de Clérambault under the term triad of automatic mental activity:

(1) automatic sensory activity (primarily hallucinations of hearing, but also sometimes of sight, smell, taste and autonomic nervous system);

(2) automatic mental activity (vocalization, reverberation, thought withdrawal, thought broadcast, and commentary on thoughts);

(3) automatic acts (subjective impression of being compelled by an outside force to move and speak);

b) delusional, most frequently persecutory, but also grandiose ideas;

c) clear sensorium, unimpaired speech, appropriate behavior and intact higher intellectual functions, contrasting sharply with the co-existing delusional and hallucinatory syndrome.

Between the two World Wars there was considerable debate in French psychiatric circles as to whether or not chronic hallucinatory psychosis constituted a legitimate diagnostic entity. In these deliberations, opposing views were propounded by de Clérambault and Henri Ey. De Clérambault, who was promptly dubbed a "mechanicist" by Ey, argued three points:

— hallucinations are caused by a diseased state of the central nervous system;

— the underlying personality plays no part in the genesis of hallucinations; the mind does not generate the hallucinatory experience but, rather, passively undergoes it;

— delusions develop secondarily and represent an attempt on the part of the intact aspects of the mind to explain the manifestations of automatic mental activity, particularly the bewildering subjective experience of hallucinations. This viewpoint is consonant with the traditional French practice of classifying delusional states according to their dominant "delusional mechanism" (in this instance, hallucinations).

For Henri Ey and the Structural(ist) School of Psychiatry he founded, hallucinations express the same meaning as the concomitant delusions, or, to put it metaphorically, hallucinations are the "voice" of delusions. If this point is conceded, then it must also be admitted that hallucinations are autonomous, and that classification should be based on the "structure" of the delusional system and of the underlying personality and not on epiphenomena, which Ey considered hallucinations to be. In 1953, Ey wrote: "There is no room for chronic hallucinatory psychosis between the two classes paranoia and schizophrenia; it straddles both."

For over 40 years the structuralists campaigned against recognition of chronic hallucinatory psychosis as a separate diagnostic entity, yet it is recognized and utilized in France: Even Ey himself devoted a highly conventional chapter to this disorder in his *Textbook of Psychiatry*.

Chronic Imaginative Psychosis

In 1911, Dupré and Logre published a series of three papers describing a new category of chronic delusional states, which they named chronic imaginative psychosis. They contended that the "imaginative mechanism" could be considered as valid a construct as the "interpretive mechanism" or the "hallucinatory mechanism." "In the hierarchy of mental operations," they wrote, "ranging from simple perceptions to the most complex beliefs or convictions . . . the delusionally imaginative individual spurns logic and the evidence of his own senses alike and expresses ideas, narrates tales and affirms facts he staunchly and unshakably believes to be true, without regard for experience or reasoning. . . . The delusionally interpretive and the delusionally imaginative individual are opposite in temperament and mental make-up: one is a reasoner, the other a rambunctious intuitive." Dupré and Logre drew a parallel with interpretive delusional states and urged that chronic imaginative psychoses be recognized on an equal footing with the other chronic delusional states. The condition they described seemed to them "to parallel chronic interpretive psychosis" in its development, symptoms and course. They stated, further, that "although the two classes of mental disorders operate with different mechanisms, both somehow seem to 'belong' to a single diagnostic class. It therefore seems to us just as logical to recognize one as it does the other, even though chronic imaginative psychosis, considered as an independent diagnosis, is assuredly far less frequently encountered in clinical practice than chronic interpretive or chronic hallucinatory psychosis."

The history of the entity chronic imaginative psychosis is complicated by the fact that Kraepelin, in the sixth edition of this textbook (1899), introduced the concept of paraphrenia, of which he described four types: systematic, expansive, confabulatory and fantastic. For Kraepelin, paraphrenias were distinguished from dementia praecox by the absence of deterioration despite a protracted clinical course. Kraepelin's paraphrenic group of 1899 and the chronic delusional states described by French clinicians between 1909 and 1911 share this common ground.

In 1920, Frey, a young Alsacian psychiatrist, attempted in his doctoral thesis to elucidate the relationship between the then current French and German classification schemes, in order to enable French psychiatrists to understand the diagnoses made by the German psychiatrists they had replaced in the psychiatric institutions of Alsace and Lorraine after peace was concluded in 1918. Frey decided that confabulatory paraphrenia could be equated with chronic imaginative psychosis, and that some cases of chronic hallucinatory psychosis could be diagnosed as fantastic paraphrenia.

Frey's attempt to establish one-to-one correspondences between the French and German classifications failed because the principles on which Kraepelin's diagnostic concepts were drafted are incompatible with the French practice of classifying disorders according to their delusional mechanism, and vice versa. Ultimately, the only diagnosis among Kraepelin's paraphrenias still recognized in French clinical practice has been fantastic paraphrenia, described by Clerc in 1925 under the name of délire fantastique* (fantastic delusional state) and considered, as it had been by Frey, to correspond to some—but not all—variants of chronic hallucinatory psychosis. In 1933, Claude suggested recognizing délire fantastique as a separate entity and calling it paraphrenia in honor of Kraepelin.**

Two significant events occurring subsequent to 1933 had repercussions on French nomenclature: First, the French structuralists gave fantastic paraphrenia a privileged position in their system, and, second, this diagnosis was reincorporated into the classificatory framework of chronic imaginative psychosis. As already pointed out, the structuralists were reluctant to classify chronic delusional states according to delusional mechanisms (it will be recalled that it was on these grounds that they had refused to recognize chronic hallucinatory psychosis in the first place). Structural theorists proposed separating chronic delusional states into three basic classes: paranoid delusional states (paranoid schizophrenia); paranoiac delusional states and paraphrenic delusional states. Schematically, this classification is based on the "structure of the delusional system," which may be coherent or incoherent, as well as on the "structure of the underlying personality," which may be diseased or intact.

In this view "paraphrenic structure" is characterized by

1) incoherent delusions, akin to a dream-like state, a feature it shares with the delusions of paranoid schizophrenia; and

2) an intact mind with unimpaired higher intellectual functions, a feature it shares with paranoia.

In addition to these two basic aspects, which define the "structure" of the disorder on two levels, two other points must be considered:

3) the fantastic, ebullient nature of the delusions; and

4) the preservation of appropriate manners and behavior which stand in contrast to the fantastic nature of the delusions.

The survival of fantastic paraphrenia as a diagnosis belonging to the class chronic delusional states results largely from the privileged position accorded to it by the structuralists, who, in theory, recognize only

---

*   Bilingual terms separated by parentheses refer to French usage where the first term is in French and the second in English, and vice versa.

** It should be noted that by this time paraphrenia had disappeared from the diagnostic vocabulary in Germany, and that the disorders to which the term originally referred had been relegated, following research that had begun with Mayer's survey in 1921, to the class paranoid schizophrenia.

two classes of (non-schizophrenic) chronic delusional states, i.e., those with paranoiac structure (the standard [intellectual] and [emotional] delusional states) and those with paraphrenic structure. Because of its two-level analytical capability, however, the structuralist system can also be used—and is used—to describe schizophrenia (see Figure 2).

Nevertheless, the structuralists did not entirely succeed in their efforts to revise French psychiatric classifications. In general, French clinicians remain attached to the diagnostic criterion of "delusional mechanisms." It is undoubtedly for this reason that chronic hallucinatory psychosis and Dupré's and Logre's chronic imaginative psychosis are still standard diagnoses in French today, and that the structuralist paraphrenic delusional states, Kraepelin's fantastic paraphrenia, Clerc's fantastic delusional state, Claude's paraphrenia and Dupré's and Logre's chronic imaginative psychosis have coalesced. The structuralists have succeeded in maintaining the term paraphrenia only for Kraepelin's fantastic variety—despite the fact that Frey had initially related the French chronic imaginative psychosis to the German confabulatory paraphrenia. This consolidation of terms was ultimately accepted by the founder of the structuralist school of psychiatry, Ey, even though, like recognition of chronic hallucinatory psychosis, it is contrary to structuralist doctrine. In the chapter of his textbook devoted to fantastic delusional states, Ey writes: "(Kraepelin's) fantastic paraphrenia is more or less congruent with chronic imaginative psychosis, isolated in France by Dupré and Logre." He lists five diagnostic criteria:

1) the fantastic nature of the delusional themes;

2) the *imaginative* (italics added) exuberance of the delusions;

3) paradoxical co-existence of a phantasmagorical subjective psychological world and good contact with reality;

4) the chaotic nature of these delusions coupled with the absence of significant mental or social deterioration;

5) the fact that higher intellectual functions remain remarkably intact.

Conclusions

The salient points of this historical review of French psychiatric diagnosis and classification may be summed up as follows:

1) From the time dementia praecox was recognized as a legitimate diagnostic class, the criterion of irreversible deterioration was consistently used in France to separate it from that class of delusional states in which deterioration does not occur. The same principle has subsequently been applied to the differentiation of schizophrenia

from the non-dissociative delusional states. As a consequence, French psychiatrists have always been careful to establish progressive and presumably permanent mental and social deterioration before diagnosing schizophrenia. This practice has resulted in the recognition of a sizeable group of non-dissociative delusional states which French clinicians view as distinct and separate from the class schizophrenia.

2) Hereditary constitution or terrain originally served as a diagnostic touchstone for transitory delusional state bouffée délirante. Although reference to the theory of degeneracy vanished around 1910, its spirit lives on in vestigial form as fragile personality, a transparent allusion to constitution or terrain still in use in France.

3) The concept of "delusional mechanisms"—interpretive, hallucinatory or imaginative—fashioned between 1909 and 1911 to differentiate between the chronic delusional states has resisted all attempts to dislodge it from diagnostic practice. It remains an intrinsic element of French diagnosis and classification.

4) No major effect has resulted from de Clérambault's attempt to draw a sharp dividing line between polarized (emotional) and non-polarized (intellectual) delusional states. In current practice, it is customary to apply this criterion only to discern between interpretive and sentimental delusional states considered as two variants of the class chronic interpretive psychosis.

5) The structuralists' campaign to substitute two-level structural description for the diagnostic device of "delusional mechanisms" has had limited impact on French diagnosis and classification. Their main achievement has been to add Kraepelin's term paraphrenia as a synonym for chronic imaginative psychosis. They have not significantly modified the French diagnostic conventions established between 1909 and 1911.

Current Views

The following survey of contemporary French approaches to psychiatric diagnosis and classification has been gleaned from: (1) the most frequently used psychiatric textbooks: Ey, Bernard and Brisset; Lemperière and Féline; Guelfi; (2) the official French classification of mental disorders published in 1968 by INSERM, Institute National de la Santé et de la Recherche Medicale (National Institute of Health and Medical Research). This classification contains no glossary, so that its diagnostic criteria cannot be reliably ascertained.

Transitory Delusional States

Transitory delusional states are considered distinct from schizophrenia by all French authors without exception. The original term transitory delusional state (bouffée délirante) has been preserved, although possible synonyms have been suggested: acute non-dissociative delusional psychoses, acute hallucinatory psychoses, oniroid or dream-like states.

Diagnostic Criteria

Current diagnostic criteria for transitory delusional state are identical to those initially suggested by Magnan (see above). The only two points diverging from Magnan's description concern causative factors and clinical course:

Causative Factors

Magnan and Legrain stated that transitory delusional states occur without (identifiable) precipitating cause or following only minimal stress. The current consensus, however, holds that, in addition to the typical and most frequent form, there are variants occasioned by psychosocial stressors, among which sudden changes in physical and emotional environment (incarceration, relocation, military service) may play a particularly important role. Although certain authors (Ey, Guelfi) relax the diagnostic criteria for transitory delusional state to include states associated with substance use and childbirth, this is not standard practice in France; the vast majority of clinicians do not consider that either post-partum psychosis or substance use disorders belong to the category transitory delusional states. On the other hand, all authors agree that there is a psychological and emotional constitution or terrain referred to as "fragile personality," a concept that has replaced Magnan's earlier term mental instability (déséquilibre mental).

Clinical Course

According to Magnan and Legrain, symptoms resolve completely in a few days to a few months. In the current view, there may be one or more episodes of transitory delusional state in the same individual (recurrent transitory delusion state), but in this case there is absolutely no sign of psychological or emotional impairment in the symptom-free intervals. Recent surveys indicate that about 40% of the psychiatric events diagnosed as transitory delusional state are non-recurrent, another approx. 40% relapse, and about 20% degenerate, following directly on the initial even or after one or more relapses, into (chronic) schizophrenia.

These two additions to Magnan's and Legrain's original views account for the diagnoses listed in the INSERM classification.

04.0 Acute or subacute delusional state presumed to be a prodromal episode of schizophrenia (accès délirant aigu ou subaigu considéré comme schizophrénique); acute schizophrenia (schizophrénie aiguë).

This diagnosis covers the 20% of events classified as transitory delusional states which will ultimately be classed as (chronic) schizophrenia. It should be noted that INSERM nomenclature does not apply the term transitory delusional state as a final diagnosis in these cases.

04.1 Acute reactive delusional psychoses (psychose délirante aiguë réactionnelle); reactive transitory delusional state (bouffée délirante réactionnelle).

These terms are used for disorders presumed to have been brought on by an identifiable psychosocial stress.

04.2 Acute delusional psychosis (psychose délirante aiguë); transitory delusional state (bouffée délirante).

Acute delusional states not classified in one of the two preceding categories.

Although the INSERM classification has no glossary, it is obvious that "genuine" transitory delusional states (i.e., those used as models in most recent French psychiatric textbooks because they conform to the pattern originally described by Magnan and Legrain) are covered by category 04.2, since they occur without identifiable precipitating cause.

INSERM 04.1 reactive transitory delusional state is mentioned in recent textbooks as a variant. There are no studies to show whether or not "genuine" transitory delusional state and reactive transitory delusional state are interrelated in any way other than through similar symptomatology and clinical course. Acute reactive delusional psychosis, which INSERM lists as a synonym for transitory delusional state, therefore seems more suitable for general use.

It would be advisable to bear in mind that the disorders described under INSERM 04.0 are not referred to as transitory delusional state.

Comparison with ICD-9 Nomenclature*

The *International Classification of Diseases* lists two diagnoses that would cover transitory delusional states:

295.4 Acute schizophrenic episode/épisode schizophrénique aigu.

The description gives criteria quite similar to those for "genuine" transitory delusional states, particularly with regard to clinical course. "In many such cases remission occurs within a few weeks or months, even without treatment." However, several essential features, such as abrupt onset and underlying fragile personality, are not mentioned. Because 295.4 disorders are viewed as a special case of schizophrenia, this entry is basically irreconcilable with transitory delusional state, which—from the French viewpoint—is always considered distinct and separate from schizophrenia.

298.3 Acute paranoid reaction (bouffée délirante).

Although this entry is designated as bouffée délirante (rendered in this chapter in English as "transitory delusional state") in the French edition of ICD-9, the diagnostic criteria describe the INSERM diagnosis bouffée délirante réactionnelle (reactive transitory delusional state). It is regrettable that the unqualified term bouffée délirante has been used in the French edition of ICD-9 for a condition which is manifestly not the disorder known in France as bouffée délirante "vraie"/"genuine" transitory delusional state; the reasons for this statement are outlined in the preceding text.

Comparison with DSM-III

The Diagnostic and Statistical Manual of Mental Disorders, Third Edition, contains no less than four diagnoses corresponding roughly to the French diagnosis transitory delusional state/bouffée délirante.

295.40 Schizophreniform disorder.

This entry describes "genuine" transitory delusional state. The only difference is that DSM-III mentions neither frequent emotional instability nor fragile personality. Nevertheless, all cases covered by DSM-III

---

*   The classification of these disorders has been significantly changed in the (draft) 10th Revision of the International Classification of Diseases (ICD-10); these differences are not discussed by the author since this chapter went to press before the new revision of the ICD was adopted (Editors).

295.40 would undoubtedly be diagnosed in France as bouffée délirante/transitory delusional state.

298.90 Atypical psychosis.

This residual category covers disorders that would be diagnosed as schizophreniform psychosis except for the fact that the condition lasts two weeks or less and that psychological stress is not mentioned as a precipitating cause. The diagnostic criteria patently describe a "genuine" transitory delusional state lasting two weeks or less. By and large, any "genuine" transitory delusional state would be covered by DSM-III diagnoses 295.40 or 298.90.

298.30 Acute paranoid disorder.

To a certain degree this diagnosis describes the reactive transitory delusional state of French nomenclature. The symptoms listed, however, do not suggest the wide-ranging variability of symptomatology viewed in France as diagnostic of all transitory delusional states, whether reactive or not.

298.80 Brief reactive psychosis.

The disorder covered by this diagnosis is the exact equivalent of the French reactive transitory delusional state which resolves in two weeks or less. Specific reference is made to predisposing factors (fragile personality).

To sum up, depending on how long the disorder persists, the "genuine" transitory delusional state recognized by French clinicians is covered either by DSM-III 295.40 or 289.90.

"Reactive" transitory delusional state lasting two weeks or less is the exact equivalent of the disorder described under 298.80. If the disorder lasts more than two weeks, it could be classified under either 298.90 or (with restrictions) 298.30.

Current Views on Chronic Delusional States

All French authors apply the conventions which separate chronic delusional states and schizophrenia into two distinct classes. Chronic delusional states are variously referred to as chronic delusional states/délires chroniques; chronic delusional psychoses/psychoses délirantes chroniques; chronic delusional syndromes/syndromes délirants chroniques and chronic non-dissociative delusional states/délires chroniques non dissociatifs.

Comparison of French and English Terminology

When discussing chronic delusional states as they are conceived of in France special care must be exercised to avoid confusion. Even though bilingual dictionaries may give the impression that the English adjectives paranoid, paranoiac and delusional are the exact equivalents of French paranoïde, paranoïaque, and délirant, French and English-speaking psychiatrists use these terms quite differently and with vastly divergent frequencies.

In France, correct technical use of the term paranoïde/paranoid is restricted to the differentiation of one form of schizophrenia. It is never appropriately used in France, as it frequently is in English-speaking countries and as its derivation would suggest, to refer to "paranoia-like" states, in other words to delusional states, which in the French view operate through a delusional mechanism of reasoning. Even further removed from French usage is the reference encountered in street talk and other loose or colloquial usage to describe feelings of uneasiness associated with (often realistic) concern over being "found out" and censured or punished. Schizophrénie paranoïde is the correct French translation of paranoid schizophrenia but there the interchangeability of the English and French terms ends; paranoid/paranoïde covers a much broader semantic field in English than it does in French.

Whereas in English it is permissible and customary to use paranoid as an adjective corresponding to the noun paranoia, the equally permissible and more precise paranoiac is only rarely used in this sense and is now practically obsolete except in substantivized forms. In France only paranoïaque/paranoiac is used to qualify paranoia-like symptoms, disorders or individuals and the use of paranoïde/paranoid for this purpose would be considered technically incorrect. To cite but one example, a paranoiac may be said to suffer from paranoid delusions in English, but only paranoiac delusions/délires paranoïques would do in French. The task of establishing equivalents or, as an ultimate aim, one-to-one correspondences between English and French nomenclature is further complicated by usage of the diagnoses paranoid states (ICD-9) and paranoid disorders (DSM-III).

Thus paranoïaque/paranoiac would definitely apply to disorders listed in ICD-9 under 297.1, probably to 297.3 and possibly to 297.0, but certainly not to 297.2. Therefore, parts of ICD-9 general class 297 are partially or totally irreconcilable with the French interpretation of paranoïaque/paranoiac, and the expression paranoid states used in the English edition of ICD-9 for 297 cannot be meaningfully construed in French nomenclature as états paranoïaques/(paranoiac states), which has narrower application.

On the other hand, since the general diagnostic criteria for entries 297.10, 297.30 and 298.30 correspond to French usages of paranoïaque/paranoiac, paranoid disorders as defined in DSM-III could probably be accurately translated into French nomenclature as troubles paranoïaques/(paranoiac disorders).

Technical French and English usages of delusional/délirant are also at variance and the two terms cannot be used interchangeably. Although it is not necessary for the purposes of this chapter to delineate the unequal semantic fields to which the term applies in France and in English-speaking countries, it should be pointed out that délirant must be used in French nomenclature to describe residual disorders described in current English usage by paranoid/paranoïde but which cannot be accurately translated into French nomenclature by either paranoïde/paranoid or by paranoïaque/paranoiac. As an example let us again consider the class of disorders grouped under 297 in the English edition of ICD-9 as paranoid disorders; in this instance the term is correctly and with technical precision rendered in the French edition as états délirants/(delusional states).

Current French Classification of Chronic Delusional States

The Broad Subdivisions

By consensus, chronic delusional states are subdivided into three broad groups: (1) chronic interpretive psychosis (also known as systematized, or paranoiac, delusional states); (2) chronic hallucinatory psychosis; (3) chronic imaginative psychosis (or paraphrenic delusional states, fantastic paraphrenias or fantastic psychoses).

Various methods have been suggested for organizing the disorders included under chronic interpretive psychosis but the distinctions usually made are trivial. The first obstacle to general agreement is difference of opinion about subdivision of chronic interpretive psychosis according to whether or not the delusional system is "polarized." De Clérambault felt it was valid to consider some delusional states polarized and others not.

INSERM classification implicitly uses polarization as a diagnostic criterion, and consequently arranges (intellectual) = interpretive + hypersensitive and (emotional) = vindicative + sentimental delusional states each on an equal hierarchical footing with the other two major subdivisions of chronic delusional states and not, as is otherwise customary, as one of the two major subdivisions of chronic interpretive psychosis (see Figures 1 and 2). This first level INSERM division of chronic delusional states can be diagrammed as follows:

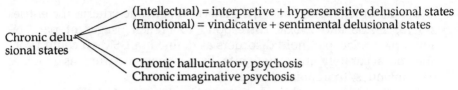

Figure 1. Classification of the chronic delusional states according to INSERM.

The remaining classifications treat interpretive and (emotional) delusional states on a par, as two subdivisions of chronic interpretive psychosis. Under this scheme, it is problematical to decide where to place Kretschmer's hypersensitive delusional state. A few authors consider hypersensitive delusional state as a major subdivision of chronic interpretive psychosis and classify it on a par with interpretive and (emotional) delusional states, while others view them simply as a subdivision of (intellectual) delusional states on a par (see Figure 2 below).

The first major subdivision is based on the criterion of "delusional mechanism" and is recognized by consensus. Opinions differ about how further to subdivide chronic interpretive psychosis. The French literature contains no specific terms recognizing this dichotomy within the class chronic interpretive psychosis although the delusional states designated in this text by the ad hoc terms (intellectual) = interpretive + hypersensitive and (emotional) = vindicative + sentimental delusional states are generally implicitly acknowledged to present broad diagnostic features by which they resemble and others by which they may be distinguished from each other. The disorders here designated as (intellectual) delusional states are called paranoiac delusional states in INSERM nomenclature. The ad hoc superordinate expression (emotional) delusional states devised for use in this chapter is referred to in French texts by the compound expression délires chroniques passionnels et de revendication. On the third divisional level, only the (Sérieux and Capgras type) interpretive and the hypersensitive delusional states define ultimate diagnostic categories; the two remaining types of disorder on this level are further subdivided into more than one clinical variant.

Fortunately, none of these organizational schemes challenge the legitimacy of either the broader classes or the ultimate diagnostic categories. One view of current French thinking about classification is reflected in Figure 2.

Classes	Genera	Species	Variants
First divisional level (by consensus)	Second divisional level: Broad class distinctions by de Clérambault following Sérieux and Capgras	Third divisional level: Sérieux and Capgras; Kretschmer; Dide and Guiraud; Kraepelin; de Clérambault	Fourth divisional level: (Sérieux and Capgras); Kretschmer; Dide and Guiraud; (Kraepelin); de Clérambault Level of specific diagnoses of variants of chronic interpretive psychosis

CHRONIC INTERPRETIVE PSYCHOSIS (STATES)

(Intellectual) delusional states[1] (not encapsulated)

Interpretive delusional states

Hypersensitive delusional states[2]

Paranoia of spinsters and governesses

Paranoia of immigrants (or of culture shock)

(Emotional) delusional states[4] (encapsulated)

Vindicative delusional states[3]

Litigious paranoia

Paranoia of social reformers and religious fanatics

Paranoia of secretive inventors

Sentimental delusional states

Conjugal paranoia

Erotic paranoia (erotomania)

CHRONIC HALLUCINATORY PSYCHOSES (STATES)

CHRONIC IMAGINATIVE PSYCHOSIS (STATES)

1) Not explicitly named in the French literature, in which they are sometimes discussed as group sharing superordinate characteristics with emotional delusional states and from which they are differentiated by some distinguishing features (see text).
2) Kretschmer's "sensitiver Beziehungswahn."
3) Akin to Kraepelin's "Querulantenwahn" or paranoia querulans
4) Not explicitly named in the French literature, in which they are sometimes discussed as sharing superordinate characteristics with intellectual delusional states and from which they are differentiated by some distinguishing features (see text).

Figure 2. A theoretical diagram of the customary French classifications of chronic delusional states, showing alternative classifications.

Differential Diagnosis of the Variants of Chronic Delusional States

Broadly speaking, chronic delusional states are differentiated from (the schizophrenic form of*) schizophrenia by the absence of mental dissociation and social deterioration (whence the occasional term non-dissociative chronic delusional states).

1. *Chronic interpretive psychosis.* As a broad class chronic interpretive psychosis is characterized by: coherent (logical) delusions; an interpretive "delusional" mechanism; the absence or inconsequentiality of hallucinations.

(Intellectual) = interpretive + hypersensitive delusional states are distinguished from (emotional) = vindicative + sentimental delusional states not only by delusional content but also according to whether the delusions remain polarized around a single theme or spread progressively to contaminate all areas of mental activity. In (intellectual) delusional states the delusional system spreads like a cancer, ultimately invading all aspects of the total outlook. In (emotional) delusional states, the delusional premise may develop in complexity but does not spread beyond the initial number of persons, groups or institutions involved in the original delusional system. For instance, in conjugal paranoia there is the delusional conviction that the spouse or lover is unfaithful. This conviction is a straightforward, stable belief and any additional interpretations only serve to enrich the original premise without spreading to other areas of the patient's mental and emotional activity, except as they relate to the original delusional premise.

As interpretive delusional states are described in standard French textbooks on psychiatry, this disorder is essentially the same as that described in other nomenclatures by the term paranoia. Because criteria are more elastic, however, the diagnosis interpretive delusional state is made with greater frequency in France than Kraepelin's paranoia vera.

Although hypersensitive delusional state was first described in Germany, this diagnosis is currently recorded with greater frequency in France. Some authors consider it a simple variant of interpretive delusional state. Distinctive features include: delusional interpretation of interpersonal relationships, a hypersensitive underlying personality (in accordance with Kretschmer's description), more frequent occurrence in certain social strata (governesses, spinsters), evidence of a precipitating event or psychosocial stressor, and an attitude of resignation towards the delusions.

---

* The apparent redundancy of the term schizophrenic form of schizophrenia acknowledges the fact that not all standard nomenclatures recognize the French distinction between schizophrenia and non-schizophrenic delusional states.

(Emotional) = vindicative + sentimental delusional states are distinguished by polarization of the basic delusional premise. They are customarily sub-divided as shown in Figure 2.

The two variants most adequately documented and described in France are: the delusional state of social reformers and religious fanatics (Dide and Guiraud), and erotic paranoia (de Clérambault).

Induced delusional state/délire induit or folie à deux is described in modern French textbooks under interpretive delusional state. Although the French term folie à deux is often employed in psychiatric textbooks written in English and other languages, this variant is never ranked as an independent diagnostic category in France.

2. *Chronic Hallucinatory Psychosis.* The diagnostic criteria currently recommended in modern French textbooks of psychiatry are practically identical to those outlined in Ballet's original description (see above).

3. *Chronic Imaginative Psychosis* (Paraphrenic delusional states, fantastic psychoses). This class is defined in modern French psychiatrist literature by diagnostic criteria derived from three sources: Dupré and Logre's original papers on chronic imaginative psychoses; Kraepelin's description of paraphrenia phantastica; and the description of paraphrenic structure found in the structural(ist) psychiatric doctrine of Claude and Ey. This type of disorder is characterized by paralogical, magical thinking; fantastic, megalomaniac delusional themes; the predominance of confabulatory over interpretive and hallucinatory delusional mechanisms; and good contact with reality contrasting sharply with extravagant delusions.

Comparison with ICD-9*

Generally speaking, the conditions known in France as chronic delusional states correspond to ICD-9 class 297 paranoid states/états délirants, insofar as the disorders belonging to this class are viewed as chronic conditions. However, there is no one-to-one correspondence between the specific disorders or variants listed under the class chronic delusional states in the French nomenclature, and the specific types of paranoid states/états délirants listed in ICD-9.

---

* The classification of these disorders has been significantly changed in the (draft) 10th Revision of the International Classification of Diseases; these differences have not been discussed by the author since this chapter went to press before the new revision of the ICD was adopted (Editors).

297.1 Paranoia.

Cases meeting the diagnostic criteria for this category would all be diagnosed in France as interpretive delusional states.

297.2 Paraphrenia.

According to the description given in the glossary, this category would appear to correspond to the French chronic hallucinatory psychosis. It should be pointed out that use of the term paraphrenia can lead to confusion as it is quite differently construed in French usage and in ICD-9. Paraphrenia as used in ICD-9 bears no relation other than phonological to the disorder bearing essentially the same name in French nomenclature.

297.3 Shared paranoid disorder/psychose induite.

As mentioned above, this disorder or dimension of a disorder is perceived in France merely as a special case or aspect of interpretive delusional state, under which it is diagnosed without further ado.

297.0 Paranoid state, simple/état délirant, forme simple.

As defined in the glossary, the French and English terms cannot be used interchangeably. Most cases meeting the diagnostic criteria for 297.0 would probably be diagnosed in France as one form or another of chronic interpretive psychosis.

To recapitulate: ICD-9 297.1, 297.3 and probably 297.0 can be correlated with chronic interpretive psychosis; ICD-9 paraphrenia corresponds to French chronic hallucinatory psychosis; ICD-9 does not define any entity even remotely connected with the meaning assigned to paraphrénie/paraphrenia in French nomenclature. Because "delusional mechanisms" constitute the foundation on which French diagnosis and classification rest and are not an explicit feature of other nomenclatures, the reliability of this tentative correlation remains moot.

Comparison with DSM-III

DSM-III contains two headings under which certain chronic delusional states could be classified.

297.10 Paranoia.

297.30 Shared paranoid disorder.

Cases covered by DSM-III 297.10 would be diagnosed in France as interpretive or possibly as one of the sentimental delusional states

(DSM-III specifies delusions of jealousy). Conditions best described under 297.30 would be diagnosed in France as interpretive delusional states. DSM-III contains no entry to which either chronic hallucinatory or chronic imaginative psychosis could be assigned.

Incidence

The following data were collected during a 1970 survey of 3,952 consecutive admissions to thirty-four French mental health facilities.

	Composition of sample	
	N	%
Dissociative		
(Chronic) schizophrenia	436	50.4
Acute schizophrenic episode		
(Acute or subacute delusional state presumed		
to be a prodromal episode of schizophrenia)	58	6.7
Nondissociative		
Transitory delusional states	149	17.2
Chronic delusional states	222	25.7
Total	865	100.0

Figure 3. Comparison of the incidence of chronic and acute schizophrenia, transitory delusional states and chronic delusional states.

	Incidence of acute psychotic episodes	
	N	%
Dissociative		
Acute schizophrenia		
(acute or subacute delusional state presumed		
to be a prodromal episode of schizophrenia)	58	28.0
Nondissociative		
Reactive transitory delusional states	38	16.5
"Genuine" transitory delusional states	115	55.5
Total	211	100.0

Figure 4. Incidence of dissociative and non-dissociative acute psychotic episodes.

The ratio of chronic delusional states to (chronic) schizophrenia is about one to two (1:2). Transitory delusional state, both "genuine" and reactive, taken together, are recorded over two and a half times as often as acute or subacute delusional state presumed to be a prodromal episode of schizophrenia.

Not only are transitory delusional states diagnosed collectively nearly three times as frequently as acute schizophrenia (or acute or subacute delusional state presumed to be a prodromal episode of schiz-

	Incidence of chronic delusional states	
	N	%
(Intellectual) delusional states	83	37.5
Chronic interpretive psychosis	98	44.1
(Emotional) delusional states	15	6.6
Chronic hallucinatory psychosis	74	33.3
Chronic imaginative psychosis	14	6.5
Unclassified	36	16.1
Total	222	100.0

Figure 5. Incidence of chronic delusional states.

ophrenia), but the "genuine" variant alone is reported more than three times as often as the "reactive" type, and twice as often as acute schizophrenia.

Arranged in order of frequency of diagnosis, the chronic delusional states are: chronic interpretive psychosis excluding (emotional) delusional states (37.5%); chronic hallucinatory psychosis (33.5%); chronic imaginative psychosis and (emotional) delusional states (6.5% each). If, as is customary, both (intellectual) and (emotional) types of chronic interpretive psychosis are combined into one class, they would account for 44% of all disorders classified broadly as chronic delusional states.

For statistical purposes, it is probably more appropriate to compare chronic delusional states to paranoid schizophrenia than to the class schizophrenia in general. This comparison is informative, as many disorders diagnosed as chronic delusional states in France would be recorded as paranoid schizophrenia in other countries.

		N		%
Dissociative				
Paranoid schizophrenia		137		38
Nondissociative				
Chronic delusional states		222		62
(Intellectual) delusional states		83		23
Chronic interpretive psychosis	98		27	
(Emotional) delusional states		15		4
Chronic hallucinatory psychosis		74		21
Chronic imaginative psychosis		14		4
Chronic delusional states not classified elsewhere		36		10
Total	222	359	62	100

Figure 6. Incidence of paranoid schizophrenia and the (non-dissociative) chronic delusional states.

Paranoid schizophrenia was diagnosed in 137 out of the total 436 cases of (chronic) schizophrenia included in this sample (31.5%).

Figure 6 gives the incidence of chronic delusional states and compares them to the total number of non-affective psychoses (= paranoid schizophrenias + chronic delusional states) in absolute numbers and percentages.

From the data included in Figures 5 and 6, it follows that chronic delusional states are diagnosed in France over one and a half times as often as paranoid schizophrenia, and that chronic interpretive psychosis is a class more widely reported in France than elsewhere. Viewed as a single broad group chronic interpretive psychosis can be considered roughly equivalent to ICD-9 297.1 and DSM-III 297.10. The disorders classified under chronic interpretive psychosis are reported in France nearly three times more often than those labelled paranoid schizophrenia. It is therefore quite evident that the diagnostic criteria applied in France to chronic interpretive psychosis are considerably more elastic than the criteria used elsewhere to classify the same or similar disorders.

Conclusions

The hallmark of French psychiatric diagnosis and classification consists of criteria restricting the diagnosis of schizophrenia and a corresponding increase in the number of non-schizophrenic delusional states reported. The statistics given in Figures 3 through 6 should be cautiously interpreted, however, as they may artificially inflate the true prevalence of both transitory and chronic delusional states. Indeed, uniform diagnostic criteria for these non-schizophrenic delusional states have never been established. More particularly, the INSERM nomenclature resorted to in the 1970 survey is an outline of diagnostic terminology without adequate discriminating definitions. This leaves extraordinary leeway for divergent diagnoses of a single disorder. If diagnostic criteria as rigorous as those in DSM-III had been established for the INSERM classification, it is most likely that far fewer cases of some non-schizophrenic delusional states would have been recorded. As a matter of fact, the prevalence of non-schizophrenic delusional states has probably been rather consistently overestimated in France. Comparison of Sérieux' and Capgras' description of interpretive delusions state to Kraepelin's paranoia vera shows that this tendency has been apparent from the beginning. The same bias is undoubtedly at work in French differentiation between transitory delusional states and acute schizophrenia. Empirical studies currently being carried out indicate that, when stringent diagnostic criteria are applied, transitory delusional states are rarely reported among new cases in French mental health facilities, whereas the statistics reported in Chapter 4 indicate that they represent about 4% of the sample population, or 154 out of 3,952 cases.

Much conjecture could be bandied about to account for this state of affairs. Historically, reluctance to accept, first, the concept of dementia praecox and, subsequently, that of schizophrenia, has been due to the incompatibility between French (particularly Magnan's) and Kraepelinian nomenclatures. Mixed transitory delusional state of degeneracy/bouffée délirante (polymorphe des dégénérés) is the only diagnosis from Magnan's classification which has survived up to the present; the diagnostic criteria of hereditary constitution on which it was originally predicated has long since been abandoned. With greater validity and more reliable criteria the differentiation of chronic delusional states was undertaken by French authors between 1909 and 1911, partly because they felt that Kraepelin's definition of paranoid schizophrenia, strictly applied, could not conceivably cover all types of delusional states and, partly because they classified disorders according to interpretive, hallucinatory or imaginative delusional mechanisms based on predominant symptoms. In France delusional mechanisms ultimately came to be considered more significant for diagnosis and classification than the delusional themes of early 19th century French nomenclature (delusions of persecution, delusions of grandeur). In the period between the two World Wars the French Structural(ist) School of Psychiatry attempted to substitute "bilevel structure" for "delusional mechanism" as a principle of diagnosis and classification. In essence, structural description is also based on predominant symptomatology and its ultimate objective is to assess the degree of organization or disorganization of the delusional system as well as of the underlying personality. In practice, however, structures have not replaced delusional mechanisms as an element of French diagnosis and classification; rather, the two concepts have merged while the classification scheme for chronic delusional states dating from the early twentieth century has remained intact.

The opinion has often been expressed that these developments have made French approaches to the diagnosis and classification of mental disorders difficult to understand. Be that as it may, opposition to Kraepelin's (and Bleuler's) nomenclature has undeniably given French psychiatry a unique stance. The striking outcome is that traditional French nomenclature reflects trends that have only recently begun to appear in other classifications. For instance, the reasoning which led to the separation of schizophreniform psychosis and atypical psychosis from schizophrenia in DSM-III resembles that which in France has kept transitory delusional state alive as a diagnostic category. The addition of still more non-schizophrenic delusional states (paranoid state, simple; paraphrenia) to ICD-9 would seem to indicate a general willingness to promote diagnosis of chronic delusional states and to abridge the scope of schizophrenia. In this respect, traditional French psychiatric concepts are highly amenable to both empirical and comparative studies, which alone can adequately assess their validity and reliability for research, as well as their usefulness for clinical practice.

APPENDIX I
BILINGUAL GLOSSARY AND SUBJECT INDEX

Explanatory Notes

Entries in **boldface print** are either psychiatric terms currently in use or the English equivalents of French terminology as translated specifically for this chapter.

Abbreviations following an entry indicate the classification system with which the term is most frequently associated: ICD-9, the *International Classification of Diseases, Ninth Revision,* published by the World Health Organization; DSM-III, *Diagnostic and Statistical Manual of Mental Disorders* (Third Edition) published by the American Psychiatric Association; INSERM, the nomenclature of the Institut National de Santé de Santé et de Recherche Médicale (National Institute for Health and Medical Research). Where no abbreviated reference follows an entry in boldface print, the term is not usually associated with any one classification system, but is rather part of modern French psychiatric vocabulary or its ad hoc equivalent in English.

Entries in *italic print* are terms of historical interest no longer in harmony with modern French psychiatric thought; such entries are followed by *obs* to indicate that they are now obsolete or obsolescent. Alternately, lightface entries are terms, such as those taken from non-French classifications, that have never been an integral part of the French psychiatric vocabulary; in this case *obs* is omitted regardless of usage.

Entries enclosed in brackets () are ad hoc terms devised specifically for the purposes of this chapter. They are designed to facilitate understanding of implicit French psychiatric concepts, discussed though not always explicitly named in the French psychiatric literature. All bracketed lightface entries relate to classification of the major subdivision of chronic interpretive psychosis, for which there is no generally recognized French classificatory convention.

Where it seems useful to give bilingual equivalents, the French term immediately follows the English; glosses are given under the entries in English and entries in French are cross-referenced to them.

Undefined entries are adequately explained in the text, and all entries referred to in the text are indexed.

Synonyms for glossary entries following any explanatory text are preceded by *syn.*

ACCES DELIRANT AIGU OU SUBAIGU CONSIDERE COMME SCHIZOPHRENIQUE, INSERM 04.0

See acute or subacute delusional state presumed to be a prodromal episode of schizophrenia.

ACUTE DELUSIONAL PSYCHOSIS/PSYCHOSE DELIRANTE AIGUE, INSERM 04

In INSERM nomenclature, class of mental disorders which includes acute schizophrenia/schizophrénie aiguë (04.0), reactive transitory delusional state/bouffée délirante réactionnelle (04.1) and "genuine" transitory delusional state/bouffée délirante "vraie" (04.2). INSERM entry 04.2 lists acute delusional psychosis as a synonym for "genuine" transitory delusional state. Use of one and same term to designate both the general class 04 and the subordinate category 04.2 is ambiguous and potentially confusing.

See acute or subacute delusional state presumed to be a prodromal episode of schizophrenia.

ACUTE OR SUBACUTE DELUSIONAL STATE PRESUMED TO BE A PRODROMAL EPISODE OF SCHIZOPHRENIA/ACCES DELIRANT AIGU OU SUBAIGU CONSIDERE COMME SCHIZOPHRENIQUE, INSERM 04.0

Diagnostic category subordinate to INSERM class 04 acute delusional psychosis/psychose délirante aiguë q.v. By definition will develop into chronic schizophrenia/schizophrénie chronique without return to premorbid level of functioning. Despite being qualified here as an acute or subacute disorder, not to be confused with transitory delusional state/bouffée délirante q.v., in which there is always a return to the premorbid level of functioning.

Syn acute schizophrenia/schizophrénique aiguë.

ACUTE HALLUCINATORY PSYCHOSIS/PSYCHOSE HALLUCINATOIRE AIGUE

See transitory delusional states.

ACUTE PARANOID DISORDER, DSM-III 298.30

ACUTE PARANOID REACTION, ICD-9 298.3

This term has been used in the English edition of ICD-9 as an equivalent of the entry bouffée délirante in the French edition. The explanatory text under ICD-9 entry 298.3, however, indicates that this diagnosis is the same as INSERM 04.1 reactive acute delusional psychosis/psychose délirante aiguë réactionnelle, that is to say, the reactive clinical form of bouffée délirante as understood in France, rather than INSERM 04.2 "genuine" transitory delusional state/bouffée délirante "vraie." Bouffée délirante as used by French psychiatrists is thus a patent misfit to the explanatory text of ICD-9 298.3. To avoid possible

confusion, reactive acute delusional psychosis/psychose délirante aiguë réactionnelle would be the best standard French term for use here.
See bouffée délirante.

REACTIVE ACUTE DELUSIONAL PSYCHOSIS/PSYCHOSE DELIRANTE AIGUE REACTIONNELLE, INSERM, 04.1
See reactive transitory delusional state.

ACUTE SCHIZOPHRENIA/SCHIZOPHRENIE AIGUE, INSERM 04.0
See acute or subacute delusional state presumed to be a prodromal episode of schizophrenia and chronic schizophrenia.

ACUTE SCHIZOPHRENIC EPISODE/EPISODE SCHIZOPHRENIQUE AIGU, ICD-9, 295.4

ATYPICAL PSYCHOSIS, DSM-III, 298.90

AUTOMATIC PERCEPTIONS
See triad of automatic mental activity.

BOUFFEE DELIRANTE (TRANSITORY DELUSIONAL STATE)
For explanation of misuse of this term in ICD-9, see acute paranoid reaction.
For INSERM classification and for current usage, see transitory delusional state.
For comparison to DSM-III, see text, page 22.

Bouffée délirante à type intermittent, obs.
See recurrent transitory delusional states.

Bouffée délirante polymorphe des dégénérés, obs.
See mixed transitory delusional state of degeneracy.

Bouffée délirante polymorphe des dégénérés à type intermittent, obs.
See recurrent mixed transitory delusional state of degeneracy.

BOUFFEE DELIRANTE REACTIONNELLE, INSERM 04.1
See reactive transitory delusional states.

BOUFFEE DELIRANTE "VRAIE"
See "genuine" transitory delusional states.

BRIEF REACTIVE PSYCHOSIS, DSM-III 298.30

CHRONIC DELUSIONAL PSYCHOSES/PSYCHOSES DELIRANTES CHRONIQUES
See chronic delusional states.

CHRONIC DELUSIONAL STATES/DELIRES CHRONIQUES

All non-schizophrenic chronic delusional states. Diagnostic class embracing all chronic delusional states not adequately defined by the French criteria for schizophrenia, i.e., those delusional states or psychoses in which progressive mental and social deterioration does not occur. Subordinate classes: in current French psychiatric usage, chronic interpretive psychosis, chronic hallucinatory psychosis, chronic imaginative psychosis; in INSERM nomenclature 0.3: (intellectual) delusional states; (emotional) delusional states; chronic hallucinatory psychosis; chronic imaginative psychosis. In modern French usage, that class of chronic psychoses not conforming to the original diagnostic canons for dementia praecox or schizophrenia and differentiated among themselves according to type of delusional mechanism q.v.; any chronic psychosis, including paranoid schizophrenia, susceptible to two-level description of delusional system and underlying personality as suggested by the French Structuralist School of Psychiatry. Derived from both senses of 2 below;

2. *obs* short for chronic delusional states of systematic evaluation q.v.; as the lines of distinction between this disorder and the chronic delusional states of degeneracy became blurred, the abbreviated form was applied indifferently to both.

Syn chronic delusional psychoses/psychoses délirantes chroniques.

Chronic delusional states of degeneracy/délires chroniques des dégénérés, obs.
See theory of degeneracy.

Chronic delusional state of systematic evaluation/délire chronique à évolution systématique, obs.
Cornerstone of Magnan's classification system.
See theory of degeneracy.
Twelve lectures on this entity were published in English by Magnan in the *American Journal of Insanity, 52.*

CHRONIC DELUSIONAL SYNDROMES/SYNDROMES DELIRANTS CHRONIQUES

See chronic delusional states.

CHRONIC EROTOMANIAC DELUSIONAL STATE/DELIRE CHRONIQUE EROTOMANIAQUE

In this chapter erotic paranoia, q.v.

CHRONIC HALLUCINATORY PSYCHOSIS/PSYCHOSE HALLUCINATOIRE CHRONIQUE, INSERM 03.2

Type of chronic delusional state defined by predominantly "delusional mechanism" q.v., to which the criteria of the triad of automatic mental activity, q.v., was subsequently added; "delusional themes" of persecution or of grandeur; absence of mental and social deterioration. See Figure 2.

CHRONIC IMAGINATIVE PSYCHOSIS/PSYCHOSE IMAGINATIVE CHRONIQUE, INSERM, 03.3

Type of chronic delusional state defined by: predominantly imaginative "delusional mechanism" q.v.; fantastically imaginative delusional themes; absence of mental and social deterioration. Historically, associated with paraphrenia. Originally described by Dupré and Logre, it was ultimately related by Frey to Kraepelin's confabulatory paraphrenia/paraphrenia confabulans. INSERM nomenclature relates this disorder to both confabulatory paraphrenia/paraphrénie confabulante and fantastic paraphrenia/paraphrénie fantastique. In current usage synonymous for all intents and purposes with the alternate chronic paraphrenic delusional state/délire chronique paraphrénique. The diagnostic criteria are: predominantly imaginative "delusional mechanism"; extravagant delusions; sharp contrast between appropriate social behavior and fantasmagorical subjective experience; disorganized delusional system; absence of mental and social deterioration: See Figure 2.

Syn chronic imagination psychosis/délire chronique d'imagination; chronic paraphrenic delusional state/délire chronique paraphrénique.

CHRONIC INTERPRETIVE PSYCHOSIS/PSYCHOSE INTERPRETATIVE CHRONIQUE

Group of chronic delusional states all of which are characterized by: predominantly interpretive "delusional mechanism" q.v.; logically coherent delusions based on the misinterpretation of correctly perceived fact(s); absence of mental and social deterioration. INSERM views this group as two differently named and distinct classes, both on a par with chronic hallucinatory and chronic imaginative psychosis, and differentiated between themselves according to whether or not the delusional core remains encapsulated or tends to spread to all areas of psychological activity. Comprises the many types of paranoia described in the French literature, including Sérieux-Capgras type interpretive delusional state, which most closely resembles Kraepelin's paranoia.

CHRONIC NON-DISSOCIATIVE DELUSIONAL STATES/DELIRES CHRONIQUES NON DISSOCIATIFS

Syn chronic delusional states, q.v.

Chronic non-hallucinatory delusional states/délires chroniques non hallucinatoires, *obs.*

Class name given by Sérieux and Capgras in 1909 to all chronic delusional states in which hallucinations were not prominent. Proceeding in this manner, they differentiated interpretive, imaginative and vindicative delusional states.

CHRONIC PARAPHRENIC DELUSIONAL STATE

See paraphrenic delusional state (chronic).

CHRONIC SCHIZOPHRENIA/SCHIZOPHRENIE CHRONIQUE

Because French psychiatric conventions restrict use of the class schizophrenia to those mental disorders that are both protracted and irreversible, it would appear that use of the term "chronic" serves here to differentiate schizophrenia as it is universally viewed in France, from the convenient but somewhat misleading French diagnosis acute schizophrenia/schizophrénie aiguë. While the symptoms for acute schizophrenia/schizophrénie aiguë, acute or subacute delusional state presumed to be a prodromal episode of schizophrenia/accès délirant aigu ou subaigu considéré comme schizophrénique, more appropriately describes the French view of schizophrenia, it is quite obviously too cumbersome for general use.

CONFABULATORY (DELUSIONAL) MECHANISM

Same as imaginative delusional mechanism.
See delusional mechanisms.

CONFABULATORY PARAPHRENIA/PARAPHRENIE
CONFABULANTE, part of INSERM 03.3

Originally described by Kraepelin as paraphrenia confabulans. Initially related in France by Frey to chronic imaginative psychosis. In INSERM nomenclature confabulatory paraphrenia, fantastic paraphrenia and chronic imaginative psychosis make up class 03.3, more generally called paraphrenic delusional state (chronic) q.v., and here called chronic imaginative psychosis, q.v.

CONJUGAL PARANOIA

See sentimental delusional states and Figure 2 above.

Constitution

See theory of degeneracy.
Constitutionally predisposed, the /prédisposés simples, *obs.*
See theory of degeneracy.

DELIRE CHRONIQUE PARAPHRENIQUE

Chronic imaginative psychosis q.v.

DELIRE CHRONIQUE PASSIONNEL, INSERM, 03.1

See emotionally delusional states.
Délire de persecution
See delusions of persecution.

DELIRE DES IDEALISTES PASSIONNES

See paranoia of social reformers and religious fanatics.

DELIRE DES INVENTEURS
See paranoia of secretive inventors.

DELIRES DES QUERULENTS PROCESSIFS
See litiginous paranoid

DELIRE D'INTERPRETATION TYPE SERIEUX ET CAPGRAS
See Sérieux-Capgras type interpretive delusional states.
Délire fantastique, *obs.*
See paraphrenia phantastica.

DELIRE INDUIT
See induced psychosis.

DELIRE INTERPETATIF, INSERM 03.0
See (intellectual) delusional states.

DELIRE PARANOIAQUE, INSERM 03.0
Chronic interpretive psychosis excluding (emotional) delusional states,
q.v.
See chronic interpretive psychosis.

DELIRE SENSITIF DE RELATION
See hypersensitive delusional states.

DELIRES
See delusions.

DELIRES CHRONIQUES
See chronic delusional states.

DELIRES CHRONIQUES NON DISSOCIATIFS
Syn chronic delusional states q.v.
Délires chroniques non hallucinatoires, *obs.*
See chronic non-hallucinatory delusional states.

DELIRES CHRONIQUES PARANOIAQUES, INSERM 03.0
See (intellectual) delusional states, for use in INSERM nomenclature
and chronic interpretive psychosis for current French usage.

DELIRES CHRONIQUES SYSTEMATISES
See chronic interpretive psychosis.

Delusional themes/thèmes du délire, obs.

DELUSIONS/DELIRES

Delusions of grandeur/délires de grandeur, obs.

DELUSIONAL/DELIRANT

Although roughly equivalent terms in bilingual dictionnaries, French- and English-speaking psychiatrists use the respective terms quite differently and with widely divergent frequencies. In French, the set délire (n)/délirant (adj.) tends to refer to a diagnostic entity, whereas the English delusion (n)/delusional (adj.) is generally limited to describing signs and symptoms and is never used in diagnoses per se; an exception to this rule, of course, is the reference to delusional states in translating French terminology in the text of this chapter. For a thorough discussion of the problems inherent in translating these terms see page 25.

DELUSIONAL MECHANISM/MECHANISMES DU DELIRE

Delusional state of degeneracy
See theory of degeneracy.

Degeneracy, obs.
See theory of degeneracy.

Degenerates, obs.
See theory of degeneracy.

Degeneration hypothesis, obs.
See theory of degeneracy.

Delusions of persecution/délires de persécution

Dementia praecox

DELIRANT
See delusional.

DELIRE A DEUX
Syn psychose induite, q.v.

Délire chronique, obs.
See chronic delusional state.

Dégénéré déséquilibré, obs.
(Unstable) degenerate. See theory of degeneracy.

Dégénéré inférieur, obs.
Inferior degenerate. See theory of degeneracy.

Dégénéré Supérieur, obs.
Superior degenerate. See theory of degeneracy.

DELIRE CHRONIQUE D'IMAGINATION, INSERM 03.3
See chronic imaginative psychosis.

DELIRE CHRONIQUE D'INTERPRETATION, INSERM 03.0
See (intellectual) delusional state.

DELIRE CHRONIQUE EROTOMANIAQUE
See erotic paranoia.

Délire chronique à évolution systématique, obs.
See chronic delusional state of systematic evolution.

DELIRE CHRONIQUE DE JALOUSIE
See sentimental delusional states and Figure 2.

DELIRE CHRONIQUE DE REVENDICATION, INSERM 03.2
See vindicative delusional states.

Dream-like states
See transitory delusional states.

Episode schizophrénique aigu
See acute schizophrenic episode.

EROTIC PARANOIA
See sentimental delusional states.
Syn chronic erotomaniac delusional state/délire chronique érotomaniaque.

EROTOMANIA
In this chapter, erotic paranoia. See sentimental delusional states.

DELIRE CHRONIQUE EROTOMANIAQUE
See erotic paranoia.

(Emotional) delusional states
(Implicit) first level major subdivisions of chronic interpretive psychosis, on a par with (also implicit) (intellectual) delusional states, q.v. Subordinate classes: vindicative and sentimental delusional states.

Encapsulation

ETATS DELIRANTS CHRONIQUES
See chronic delusional states.

Etats paranoïaques
See paranoid disorders.

Expansive paraphrenia

ETAT DELIRANT, FORME SIMPLE
See paranoid state, simple.

ETAT ONIROIDE
See transitory delusional states.

ETATS DELIRANTS, ICD-9 297
See paranoid states.

FOLIE A DEUX, ICD-9 297.3
Syn for ICD-9 entry induced psychosis q.v.

Folie des dégénérés, obs.
See delusional states of degeneracy.

Fantastic delusional states/délires fantastiques
See paraphrenia phantastica and chronic imaginative psychosis.

FANTASTIC PARAPHRENIA/PARAPHRENIE FANTASTIQUE, INSERM 03.3
See paraphrenia phantastica and chronic imaginative psychosis.

FANTASTIC PSYCHOSIS/PSYCHOSE FANTASTIQUE
Same as paraphrenic delusional state (chronic) q.v. or (here) chronic imaginative psychosis q.v.

Hypersensitive delusional states
One level in the step-like subdivision of chronic interpretive psychosis. Subordinate diagnoses: paranoia of spinsters and governesses; paranoia of culture shock. Superordinate class: (intellectual) = interpretive + hypersensitive delusional states. See Figure 2.
Syn (Kretschmer's) sensitiver Beziehungswahn, reference paranoia.

INDUCED DELUSIONAL STATES/DELIRE INDUIT
See induced psychosis.

INDUCED PSYCHOSIS/PSYCHOSE INDUITE, ICD-9 297.3
Classed under chronic interpretive psychosis, not considered in France to constitute an autonomous diagnostic category (in current French usage).
Syn induced delusional state/délire induit and (shared insanity/folie à deux).

FORME SCHIZOPHRENIQUE DE LA SCHIZOPHRENIE
See schizophrenic form of schizophrenia.

Fragile personality
See theory of degeneracy.

"Genuine" transitory delusional states/bouffée(s) délirante(s) "vraies"

(INTELLECTUAL) DELUSIONAL STATES

Used in this chapter to designate INSERM class 03.0 in English. (Implicit) first level major subdivision of chronic interpretive psychosis, on a hierarchical par with (emotional) delusional states, q.v., used here for INSERM class 03.10. Subordinate classes: interpretive (no further explicit subdivision) and hypersensitive delusional states q.v. The immediately superordinate class in this chapter is chronic interpretative psychosis; the immediately superordinate class in INSERM nomenclature is chronic delusional states. See Figure 2.

INTERPRETIVE DELUSIONAL STATES

Most frequent ultimate diagnosis under the class chronic interpretive psychosis. The diagnostic criteria are most elastic than those for paranoia, with which it is practically synonymous. No clearly defined subordinate diagnoses. Superordinate class: (intellectual) = interpretive + hypersensitive delusional states; diagnostic criteria: multiple, logically interrelated delusional themes; absence or inconsequentiality of hallucinations; lucid thought; web-like progression of delusional thinking; unimpaired social behavior, except as motivated by the delusional system. Originally described by Sérieux and Capgras. Together with hypersensitive delusional states, constitutes INSERM class 03.0, which is referred to in this chapter as (intellectual) delusional states. See Figure 2.

Involuntary acts
See triad of automatic mental activity.

Inferior degenerate/dégénéré inférieur
See theory of degeneracy.

INSERM

Délires chroniques 03
Délires chroniques paranoïaques or délire chronique d'interprétation 03.0
Délire chronique passionnel et de revendication 03.1
Délire hallucinatoire chronique 03.2
Délire chronique paraphrénique 03.3
Non-dissociative delusional states

ONIROID STATES/ETAT ONIROIDE

One of the terms suggested by several contemporary French authors to replace transitory delusional state/bouffée délirante in French nomenclature.
See transitory delusional states.
Recurrent mixed transitory delusional states of degeneracy/bouffée

délirante polymorphe des dégénérés à type intermittent, *obs.*
Relapsing form of mixed transitory delusional state of degeneracy, q.v. in which there is a documented history of one or more episodes separated by completely symptom-free intervals.

LITIGIOUS PARANOIA/DELIRE DES QUERULENTS PROCESSIFS
See vindicative delusional states and Figure 2.

Mixed transitory delusional state of degeneracy/bouffée délirante polymorphe des dégénéré, obs.
Diagnostic category defined by Magnan and Legrain. The original diagnostic criteria remain practically unchanged in current French psychiatric practice. Also variously known as: transitory delusional state/bouffée délirante q.v. transitory delusional state of degeneracy/bouffée délirante des dégénérés; "genuine" transitory delusional state/bouffée délirante "vraie" (type Magnan).

Mechanicist School of Psychiatry

PARANOIA OF SECRETIVE INVENTORS/DELIRE DES INVENTEURS
See vindicative delusional states and Figure 2.

PARANOIA OF SOCIAL REFORMERS AND RELIGIOUS FANATICS/DELIRE DES IDEALISTES PASSIONNES
See vindicative delusional states and Figure 2.

PARANOIA OF SPINSTERS AND GOVERNESSES
See hypersensitive delusional states.

REACTIVE TRANSITORY DELUSIONAL STATES/BOUFFEE DELIRANTE REACTIONNELLE, INSERM 04.1
Diagnosis applied to disorders manifesting the same signs and symptoms as "genuine" transitory delusional state/bouffée délirante vraie" q.v. but related to a documented psychosocial stressor. This diagnosis is made less frequently than "genuine" transitory delusional state and is now viewed by most French clinicians as variant of transitory delusional state q.v.
Syn acute reactive delusional psychosis/psychose délirante aiguë réactionelle.

PARANOIA, ICD-9 297.1, DSM-III 297.10
Although this term had previously been employed to describe delusions of persecution, jealousy, etc., it was given its present definition by Kraepelin. Although it is commonly used in France, French-speaking psychiatrists are more likely to use the generic terms chronic paranoiac delusional states q.v. as in INSERM nomenclature, or chronic systematized delusional states, q.v. of general usage, both of which cover a

wider range of mental disorders than paranoia in the strict sense of the word.

PARANOIA OF CULTURE SHOCK/PARANOIA SENSITIVE DES ETRANGERS

See hypersensitive delusional states.

PARANOIAC DELUSIONAL STATES (CHRONIC)/DELIRES (CHRONIQUES) PARANOIAQUES, INSERM 03.0

In INSERM nomenclature, one of the four subdivisions of chronic delusional states. Includes interpretive and hypersensitive but excludes vindicative and sentimental delusional states. In current French psychiatric usage, this term is employed synonymously with systematized delusional states (chronic)/délires (chroniques) systématisés q.v. Throughout this chapter chronic interpretive psychosis has been used and, where necessary to make the INSERM distinction, a qualifying phrase has been added, e.g. chronic interpretive psychosis excluding (emotional) delusional states. See Figure 2.

Paranoiac structure, obs.

According to the French Structuralist School of Psychiatry, one of the three basic types of two-level structure of chronic delusional states (here only) including schizophrenia. In it delusions are well organized and the underlying personality intact. It applies to systematized (or paranoiac) delusional states or those disorders classed here under chronic interpretive psychosis.

PARANOIAQUE

See paranoiac.

PARANOIA SENSITIVE, INSERM 03.0

Here called hypersensitive delusions states q.v.
Syn délire sensitif de relation.

PARANOIA VERA

PARANOIAC/PARANOIAQUE

In France, adjective corresponding to the noun paranoia, which is never modified by paranoid; or used as a substantivized adjective for anyone suffering from paranoia. It is generally applicative to any of the disorders classified here under the term chronic interpretive psychosis q.v.

PARANOID STATES/ETATS DELIRANTS, ICD-9 297

Both the English and the French, though disparate in origin, apply equally well to ICD-9 class 297.

Paranoid structure, obs.
According to the French Structuralist School of Psychiatry, one of the three basic types of two-level structure of chronic delusional states (here only) including schizophrenia. It features a disorganized delusional system and a deteriorating underlying personality. It applies to paranoid schizophrenia.

PARANOIDE
See paranoid.

PARANOID/PARANOIDE
The English variously translates to French paranoïde, paranoïaque or délirant. English paranoid is used much more loosely and frequently than French paranoïde, which is employed only to differentiate one type of schizophrenia.

PARANOID DISORDERS, DSM-III
Diagnostic class embracing both chronic delusional states, paranoia and shared paranoid disorders as well as one acute delusional state, acute paranoid disorder. May in some instances be translated into French by états paranoïaques (paranoiac states).

PARANOID STATE, SIMPLE/ETAT DELIRANT, FORME SIMPLE ICD-9 297.0
Both the English and the French apply equally well to ICD-9 297.0.

Paraphrenia confabulans, obs.
One of Kraepelin's variants of paraphrenia q.v.
See also confabulatory paraphrenia.

Paraphrenia expansiva, obs.
One of Kraepelin's variants of paraphrenia q.v.

Paraphrenia phantastica, obs.
One of Kraepelin's variants of paraphrenia q.v. Diagnostic category for which Clerc suggested the French term délire fantastique to be used for diagnosis and classification of chronic hallucinatory psychosis.

Paraphrenia
1. Class briefly differentiated from dementia praecox by Kraepelin because deterioration (dementia) did not occur, then reabsorbed into the original class *obs*;
2. An entry in ICD-9, 297.2. The diagnostic criteria describe the French chronic hallucinatory psychosis q.v. and not (chronic) paraphrenic delusional state q.v. Therefore, use of this term to head diagnosis 297 in the French edition of ICD-9 is questionable;
3. The Structuralist School attempted to honor Kraepelin by substitut-

ing paraphrenia for Clerc's fantastic delusional state;
4. Abbreviation for (chronic) paraphrenic delusional state q.v.

PARAPHRENIA, ICD-9 297.2

Paraphrénie, obs.
Name given by Claude's School to Clerc's fantastic delusional
state/délire fantastique q.v. in honor of Kraepelin. Later, Ey's Structuralist School derived from it the concept "paraphrenic structure" q.v.
that is, a loosely structured delusional system and an unimpaired underlying personality. Correctly, paraphrénie serves as an abbreviation
for délire chronique paraphrénique.

PARAPHRENIE, ICD-9 297.2

PARAPHRENIE FANTASTIQUE, INSERM 03.3

Paraphrenia Systematica, obs.
One of Kraepelin's variants of paraphrenia q.v.

PARAPHRENIC DELUSIONAL STATE (CHRONIC)/DELIRE (CHRONIQUE) PARAPHRENIQUE

Same as chronic imaginative psychosis q.v.
Syn fantastic psychosis.

Paraphrenic structure, obs.
According to the French Structuralist School of Psychiatry one of the
three basic types of two-level structure of chronic delusional states
(here only) including schizophrenia. Characterized by disorganized
delusional system and unimpaired underlying personality. Applies to
chronic imaginative psychosis, also known as paraphrenic delusional
states, (chronic).

PERSONALITE FRAGILE

See fragile personality.

PSYCHOSES DELIRANTES AIGUES, INSERM 04

See acute delusional psychosis.

PSYCHOSE DELIRANTE AIGUE REACTIONNELLE, INSERM 04.1

See reactive acute transitory delusional state

PARAPHRENIE CONFABULANTE, INSERM 03.3

Paraphrenias, the, obs.

Predispose simple, obs.
See constitutionally predisposed.
Syn sujet à prédisposition latente.

PSYCHOSE INDUITE
See induced psychosis.

PSYCHOSE IMAGINATIVE CHRONIQUE
See chronic imaginative psychosis.

PSYCHOSE INTERPRETATIVE CHRONIQUE
See chronic interpretive psychosis.

PSYCHOSE FANTASTIQUE
See fantastique psychosis.

PSYCHOSES HALLUCINATOIRE AIGUE
See acute hallucinatory psychosis and transitory delusional states.

PSYCHOSE HALLUCINATOIRE CHRONIQUE, INSERM 03.2
See chronic hallucinatory psychosis.

SCHIZOPHRENIC FORM OF SCHIZOPHRENIA/FORME SCHIZOPHRENIQUE DE LA SCHIZOPHRENIE
Apparent redundancy, which underscores the French view, sharply contrasting schizophrenia with non-dissociative chronic delusional states, in which mental and social deterioration, in contradistinction to the French concept of schizophrenia, does not occur or is minimal.

SCHIZOPHRENIE AIGUE, INSERM 04.0
See acute schizophrenia.

SCHIZOPHRENIE CHRONIQUE
See chronic schizophrenia.

PSYCHOSES DELIRANTES CHRONIQUES
Syn chronic delusional states q.v.

Querulantenwahn, obs.
Kraepelin, Akin to vindicative delusional states as used here.

Schizophrenia

SHARED PARANOID DISORDER, DSM-III 297.30

Shared paranoid state

Stigmata of degeneracy, obs.
See theory of degeneracy.

SCHIZOPHRENIFORM DISORDER, DSM-III 295.40

SENTIMENTAL DELUSIONAL STATES
One level (penultimate) in the step-like subdivisions of class chronic interpretive psychosis. Subordinate diagnoses: conjugal paranoia;

erotic paranoia. Superordinate class: INSERM 03.1 here called (emotional) = vindicative + sentimental delusional states. See Figure 2.

SERIEUX-CAPGRAS TYPE INTERPRETIVE DELUSIONAL STATES

Usual designation for the mental disorders described outside of France as paranoia. Named for the authors who described paranoiac states according to their "delusional mechanism" q.v., thus rendering diagnostic criteria for this condition more flexible in France than elsewhere. See interpretive delusion states and Figure 2.

Structure Paraphrenique, obs.
See paraphrenic structure.

Sujet à prédisposition latente, obs.
Constitutionally predisposed.
See theory of degeneracy.

Superior degenerates, obs.
See theory of degeneracy.

Structuralist School of Psychiatry

Structure paranoïaque, obs.
See paranoiac structure.

Structure paranoïde, obs.
See paranoid structure.

SYSTEMATIZED OR PARANOIAC DELUSIONAL STATES/DELIRES SYSTEMATISES OU PARANOIAQUES

A combination of INSERM nomenclature and current French psychiatric usage. INSERM calls this class of interpretive delusional states (chronic) paranoiac delusional states/délires chroniques paranoïaques and includes under it interpretive and hypersensitive delusional states but not vindicative and sentimental delusional states.

Terrain
See theory of degeneracy.

Thèmes du délire
See delusional themes.

SYNDROMES DELIRANTS CHRONIQUES

Syn chronic delusional states q.v.

SYSTEMATIZED DELUSIONAL STATES (CHRONIC)/DELIRES (CHRONIQUES) SYSTEMATISES

Synonymous with chronic interpretive psychosis which has been used throughout this Chapter. In current French psychiatric usage, paranoiac delusional states (chronic)/délires (chroniques) paranoïaques is a synonym. However, here the term does not serve the same superordinate function as INSERM's paranoic delusional states (chronic) q.v. In current French psychiatric usage, the term (chronic) paranoiac delusional states is used interchangeably with (chronic) systematized delusional states/délires chroniques systematsés; although it includes the same entities as INSERM, it is subdivided into three subordinate classes: interpretive, hypersensitive and (emotional) = vindicative + sentimental delusional states. These two approaches to the classification of the chronic interpretive psychosis is laboriously erased by using the cumbersome expression systematized or paranoiac delusional states. In this chapter, the less ambiguous class term chronic interpretive psychosis, more consistent with the other appellations of categories also subordinate to chronic delusional states, has been consistently used throughout. Where necessary to indicate one particular usage or another, an explanatory phrase has been added, e.g., chronic interpretive psychosis excluding (emotional) delusional states.

Triad of automatic mental activity/triple automatisme mental, obs.

Under this expression de Clérambault arranged the psychopathological features of chronic hallucinatory psychosis; automatic perceptions = hallucinations; automatic mentation = thought diffusion; automatic acts = subjective impression of being compelled to speak and move by an outside force.

Triple automatisme mental, obs.

See triad of automatic mental activity.

TRUE TRANSITORY DELUSIONAL STATE

See "genuine" transitory delusional state and transitory delusional state.

Theory of degeneracy, obs.

Refers to Morel's hypothesis or Magnan's clinical version of it. The keystone to Magnan's classification was the diagnosis chronic delusional state of systematic evolution, q.v. He erroneously believed the bulk mental disorders he observed were the same clinical entity, diverging in presentation only because they were seen at different stages in their clinical course. He ingeniously accounted for mental disorders patently not accommodated by the protean chronic delusional state of systematic evolution by applying the theory of degeneracy to his constructs or, more accurately, his constructs to the interpretation of the theory. Chronic delusional states running an exemplary clinical course were taken as a sign of normal hereditary constitution, while mental disorders of variance with the criteria for chronic delusional states were considered to prove an underlying degenerate genotype and to demonstrate that the individuals in which they occurred were degenerates. Following his ideas to their logical conclusion, he stated that intellectually limited individuals (idiots, imbeciles, morons) were inferior degenerates, and that any mental disorder they displayed belonged to a special diagnostic class; intellectually normal individuals not exhibiting the diagnostic signs of chronic delusional states when mentally ill were thus superior degenerates demonstrating their deficient heredity in sickness, and their mental disorders belonged to a distinct diagnostic class.

TRANSITORY DELUSIONAL STATE/BOUFFEE DELIRANTE, INSERM 04.2 and popular usage.

Short for mixed transitory delusional state of degeneracy/bouffée délirante, polymorphe des dégénérés, as originally described by Magnan and Legrain. The modifier "genuine" or "idiopathic" is used to distinguish between essential or true transitory delusional state/bouffée délirante "vraie" and reactive transitory delusional state/bouffée délirante réactionnelle. Diagnostic criteria: sudden onset; absence of identifiable precipitating cause; jumbled, shifting delusional themes; variability of delusional material; (frequent) confusion; (frequent) emotional instability; (frequent) hallucinations; no repercussions on general health; rapid and complete remission with return to premorbid level of functioning; underlying fragile personality; single episode or recurring episodes alternating with symptom-free intervals. *Syn* oniroid state/état oniroïde.

Transparency of thoughts
See triad of automatic mental activity.

VINDICATIVE DELUSIONAL STATES/DELIRE CHRONIQUE DE REVENDICATION, INSERM 03.1

Group of chronic delusional states featuring an interpretive "delusional mechanism" and sharing the differentiating diagnostic criterion of encapsulation q.v. with sentimental delusional states q.v.; because vindicative and sentimental delusional states both exhibit encapsulation they are often considered one superordinate class for which the contrived term (emotional) delusional states q.v. has been used in this text. There is no explicit French term for this broad order of conditions, but where necessary for discussing them, the French use the component parts together to designate the broader class as vindicative and sentimental delusional states/délires chroniques passionnels et de revendication. Vindicative delusional states were introduced as a concept in French psychiatry at about the same time as Kraepelin's Querulantenwahn. See Figure 2.

VINDICATIVE DELUSIONAL STATES/DELIRES CHRONIQUES DE REVENDICATION, INSERM 03.1

One level penultimate in the step-like subdivision of class chronic interpretive psychosis. Subordinate diagnoses: litigious paranoia; paranoia of social reformers and religious fanatics; paranoia of secretive inventors. Superordinate class (Emotional) = vindicative + sentimental delusional states. See Figure 2.

APPENDIX II
References

The references listed below are limited to the bare minimum required to document the main points made in this chapter. Some are typewritten doctoral theses to be found only in the libraries of the medical schools where they are on deposit.

On Magnan's theories:

Magnan, V. and M. Legrain: Les Dégénérés (Etat mental et syndromes épisodiques). Paris: Rueff et Cie., 1895.

and more generally

Magnan, V. Leçons cliniques sur les maladies mentales. Paris: Louis Bataille, 1893 (second edition).

The keystone of Magnan's theories, Délire chronique à évolution systématique/chronic delusional state of systematic evolution, is described in:

Magnan, V. and P. Sérieux. Le délire chronique à évolution systématique. Paris: Gauthier Villars/Georges Masson, 1893.

An accurate and well documented review of Magnan's ideas on pathogenesis is given in:

Genil-Perrin, G. Histoire des origines et de l'évolution de l'idée de dégénéréscence en médecine mentale. Paris: Alfred Leclerc, 1913 (doctoral thesis).

The original description of bouffées délirantes/transitory delusional states is found in:

Legrain, M. Du délire chez les dégénérés. Paris: Librairie A. Deshaye et E. Lecrosnier, 1886 (doctoral thesis)

Two important general reviews are included in:

Dublineau, J. Les bouffées délirantes; revue générale. Semaine des hôpitaux, 1932, (1), 25-30.

Appia, O. Evolution de la notion de bouffée délirante polymorphe dans la psychiatrie française depuis Magnan jusqu'à nos jours. Paris: Dactylo-Sorbonne, 1964 (doctoral thesis).

The original description of Délire d'interpretation (Sérieux-Capgras type paranoia) is:

Sérieux, P. and J. Capgras. Les folies raisonnantes. Le délire d'interprétation. Paris: Félix Alcan, 1909. (See review of this book in English in: American Journal of Insanity, Vol. LXVI, p. 182)

A penetrating analysis of trends between the two World Wars is given in:

Sérieux, P. and J. Capgras. Délires systematisés chroniques in E. Sergent, L. Ribadau-Dumas, and L. Babonneix (eds.) Traité de pathologie médicale et de thérapeutique appliquée. VII. Tome I. Psychiatrie. Paris: Maloine 1926 (second edition), 233-311.

G. de Clérambault's concepts of erotic and conjugal paranoia are described in a series of papers collected in:

Clérambault, G. de. Oeuvre psychiatrique. Paris: Presses Universitaires de France, 1942 (2 vols).

The original description of chronic hallucination psychosis is found in:

Ballet, G. La psychose hallucinatoire chronique. Encéphale, 1911, 401-411.

Ballet, G. La psychose hallucinatoire chronique et la désagrégation de la personalité. Encéphale, 1913, 501-508.

A subsequent classical description is given in:

Sérieux, P. and J. Capgras. Délires systématisés chroniques. op. cit.

The most recent overview is:

Dalle, B. Les syndromes hallucinatoires idiopathiques chroniques de l'adulte. Lille, 1964 (doctoral thesis).

Chronic imaginative psychosis was originally described in:

Dupré, E. and L. Logre. Les délires d'imagination. Mythomanie délirante. Encéphale, 1911, 209-232; 337-350; 430-450.

The classical subsequent description is:

Sérieux, P. and J. Capgras. Délires systématisés chroniques. op. cit.

The theories of the Structuralist School of Psychiatry were first published in:

Nodet, C. Le groupe des psychoses hallucinatoires chroniques. Paris: Doin, 1937.

The complex historical relations between imaginative delusional states and Kraeplin's paraphrenias are reviewed in:

Bridgman, F. Le groupe des paraphrénies dans ses rapports avec la classification française des troubles mentaux. Paris: Dupuytren-Copy, 1972 (doctoral thesis).

Current French nomenclature is reflected in:

Encyclopedie médicochirurgicale, psychiatrie clinique et thérapeutique (3 vols.). Paris: Editions Techniques (published periodically).

Ey, H., Bernard, P. and C. Brisset. Manuel de Psychiatrie. Paris: Masson et Cie, 1974 (fourth edition).

Guelfi, J. Eléments de psychiatrie. Paris: Editions médicales et universitaires, 1979 (second edition).

Lemperière, T. and A. Féline. Psychiatrie de l'adulte. Paris: Masson 1977.

The full title of the official French nomenclature published by INSERM is:

Institut National de la Santé et de la Recherche Médicale. Section psychiatrie: Classification française des troubles mentaux. Paris 1968. Bulletoin de l'Institut National de la Santé et de la Recherche Médicale. 24, 1969. Supplement to No. 2.

Standard nomenclatures used for purposes of comparison:

International Classification of Diseases, Ninth Revision, Vol. 1 (1975). World Health Organization. Geneva, Switzerland, 1977 (ICD-9).

Diagnostic and Statistical Manual of Mental Disorders, Third Edition. Washington, D.C., American Psychiatric Association, 1980 (DSM-III).

Mental Disorders: Glossary and Guide to their Classification in Accordance with the Ninth Revision of the International Classification of Diseases. Geneva, World Health Organization, 1978 (ICD-9).

The incidence of disorders in France is taken from:

Pichot, P. and H. Debray. Hospitalisation psychiatrique. Statistique descriptive. Paris: Sandoz Editions, 1971.

3
Psychiatric Diagnosis in the German-Speaking Countries

J. Glatzel*

An account of current practice in diagnosis and classification of psychiatric disorders in the German-speaking countries demands an outline of its scientific-historical background and a description of the main trends and streams of psychiatric and psychological thought in relation to the separate groups of disorders, viz., those of the endogenous psychoses, the organic disorders, the abnormal personalities and neurosis, gerontopsychiatry, and the mental disorders of childhood and adolescence.

The Endogenous Psychoses

The Schizophrenias

Historical Outline

Recent discussions on the concept of schizophrenia in the German-speaking countries can be traced back to the era of late romanticism when the theory of unitary psychosis evolved.

The concept of unitary psychosis is connected above all with Zeller and Griesinger, although the latter abandoned it in the late years of his life. It reflects the spirit of the era of romanticism, i.e., the search for a way out of a "split world" back to unity and identity in all fields, as well as the attempt to explain all functions of life and their interdependence as expressions of an obscure totality.

Zeller's teaching on unitary psychosis is based on two important premises. First, he opposed the idea that mental diseases should be regarded as primary diseases of the brain. Far from overlooking the

* Forensische Psychiatrie, Klinikum der Universität, 6500 Mainz, Federal Republic of Germany.

dependence of mental life upon its organic basis, he stressed the common origin of Psyche and Bios. It is not that humans consist of body and soul; rather, they are a body and a soul simultaneously. All mental diseases spring from a common basis, which he called "the pain of the soul" (Seelenschmerz), the "painful spirit of the inner." Together with the theory of the common origin of all mental diseases, of all the stages it is the one that is of greatest importance to the notion of unitary psychosis. According to it, the so-called basic forms of madness should not be regarded as separate diseases, but as stages in the course of a single disease. These stages are: sadness (Schwermut), i.e., melancholia, raving madness (Tollwut) and mania; mental derangement (Verrücktheit), frenzy insanity (Wahnsinn), paranoia and lunacy (Wahnwitz) as well as imbecility (Blödsinn), amentia and dementia, in various forms and degrees of presentation.

The doctrine of the stages as an important element in the teaching of unitary psychosis was soon abandoned in the clinic and has only recently been revived. Griesinger, in 1861, classified the idiopathic mental disorders into four forms of illness: melancholia, mania, derangement and imbecility.

Snell's concept of the "primary syndromes" (primäre Syndrome), dating from 1865, denoted by himself and other authors as Wahnsinn (insanity), inevitably led to a new diagnostic orientation, inasmuch as the clinical pictures described by Snell were considered until then to be merely secondary mental impairments. Westphal enlarged the spectrum of symptoms of Snell's "insanity" (Wahnsinn) in 1878, and this provided the basis for Janzarik's statement in 1980 that it was Westphal who established the convention on schizophrenia largely accepted in a later period. The diagnostic situation on the eve of Kraepelin's era could be summarized as follows: Snell and Westphal had already described the predominately delusional paranoid psychoses as primary mental derangements; Kahlbaum had delineated catatonia in 1883; and Hecker, commissioned by Kahlbaum, had presented hebephrenia in 1871. Finally, the blunt dementia simplex resulting in mental deficiency was described 30 years later by Diem under the title *The Simple Dement Form of Dementia Praecox (Dementia Simplex)* (1903). The "Heboidophrenia" typified by Kahlbaum in 1884 was generally recognized only for a short time; the case descriptions published by Hecker and himself later, in an attempt to illustrate the "heboid," give the idea rather of abnormal and psychopathic personalities.

Kraepelin then grouped those allegedly separate illnesses under a larger notion for which he called "dementia praecox," a term he took over from Morel. He considered them to be one disease entity, modelled upon general paresis and presumably characterized by a common cause, a common somatic and mental symptomatology, a common course and common autopsy findings. From the sixth edition of his textbook (1899) onwards, dementia praecox was juxtaposed to the other mental disease, manic-depressive illness. Kraepelin's nosology was accepted in its original form for only a relatively short time; he himself radically questioned it in a famous treatise of 1920. Nevertheless, K. Schneider's statement in one of his discourses in 1955: "Kraepelin's era has not yet come to an end. The piles erected by him are still standing" is still valid for part of the psychiatry of the German-speaking countries.

It was mostly Jaspers, Gruhle and K. Schneider who, on the one hand, complemented and strengthened the psychopathological foundations of Kraepelin's nosological system and, on the other, modified it in such a way to ensure its use up to the present. They drew the necessary conclusions from a development threatening to lead psychiatric doctrine into a dead end by orienting it rigidly toward the paresis model, i.e., a strictly naturalistic viewpoint. Jaspers, followed by Gruhle, resolved the impossibility of determining the diagnosis of dementia praecox somatically by demanding its differentiation from non-psychotic disturbances on a purely psychological level. Jaspers differentiated between a qualitative mental abnormality—necessarily psychotic and thus biologically based—and a quantitative abnormality—optionally psychotic and thus optionally biological; he made a strong effort in a paper (still appreciated) to differentiate between personality development and its process-like destruction. After the Kraepelinean notion of dementia praecox was replaced by Bleuler's term "schizophrenia"—mainly prognostically neutral—it was K. Schneider who, in his *Clinical Psychopathology*, outlined, in his own words, the differential typology of endogenous mental diseases, describing as well three types of schizophrenia: paranoid, simple and catatonic. (He explicitly excluded the hebephrenias because in his view they did not constitute a separate type, but were characterized by age of onset of illness alone.) Later Huber added to those types the coenesthetic one (first published 1953). K. Schneider drew as sorts of diagnostic guidelines from the manifold psychopathological facts the symptoms of the first and the second rank. He noted that those of the first rank made it possible to speak of schizophrenia provided only that there was no organic, i.e., symptomatic, psychosis, as evidenced by the absence of clouded consciousness. K. Schneider's *Clinical Psychopathology*, its last edition revised by him appearing in 1967, marks the preliminary end of the dominantly naturalistic psychiatric doctrine in the German-speaking countries. Other trends of thought, hardly heard of for a long time, now moved closer to the scene.

Before going on to them, brief mention should be made of those authors who tended to follow Kraepelin's biological concept. They belonged to the school of Kleist, inherited later by Leonhard, who endeavored to delineate a number of separate clinical pictures out of the group of schizophrenia in order to describe them as independent nosological entities, kinds of heredogenerative illnesses. However, his proposal for a *Subdivision of Endogenous Psychoses* (1959) raised little interest—although some of his newly introduced or revived terms survived with a different content.

The Concept of Schizophrenia

In the early 1950s widespread efforts were made to de-emphasize the traditional concept of schizophrenia, enabling investigators to redis-cover and further develop certain notions arrived at as early as the 1920s. They were driven by mistrust in the conviction inherited from the last quarter of the 19th century that psychiatry—analogous to other branches of medicine—was obliged to follow a strictly naturalistic mode of thinking.

Klaus Conrad, whose monograph *The Initial Schizophrenia* was preceded by a number of important publications, especially on the subject of aphasia, opened the way for Gestalt psychology to gain access mainly to the psychopathology of delusions. A few years earlier, Matussek (1952/53) had presented fundamental contributions to the research of delusional perception using the same methods. Conrad's and Matussek's investigations were relevant to the doctrine on schizo-phrenia mainly because of their effort to substitute for the division of this endogenous psychosis into separate, relatively independent, sub-types a unitary interpretation of schizophrenic illness considered as different stages of the course of a single disease process. Later Janzarik (1968) named the presumably distinct subforms of schizophrenia "in-stant photographs of a continuum" and denied the diagnostic impor-tance of such concepts as simple, paranoid-hallucinatory, catatonic and other categories of schizophrenia. Conrad's monograph contains anoth-er important idea: He claimed that the classical schizophrenic symp-toms were of little importance for grasping the "virtue" or the "essence" of the disease, by attributing a specific schizophrenic quality to the reduction of the mental potential, considering this a specific feature of schizophrenic disorders. His quest for a basic disturbance, a basic symptom, provided a link to some investigations in the early 20th century (e.g., the "primary symptoms" of E. Bleuler (1926), and the "basic symptoms" of Berze (1914), Kronfeld (1922)). In terms of his strictly somatological attitude, Conrad understood the reduction of potential as a mainly biologically determined mental abnormality. He attempted to replace the relatively rigid subdivision of the forms of schizophrenic illness by a unitary concept of variously manifested schizophrenia—while at the same time preserving the Kraepelinean dichotomy. And his efforts to translate Schneider's criteria into the language of modern psychology are nowadays reflected in the work of Janzarik, Kisker and Petrilowitsch. Janzarik outlined a structural-dy-namic concept of schizophrenic psychoses (e.g., 1959, 1968). Kisker applied the topological psychology of Lewin, and Petrilowitsch the structural psychology of Krueger and Welleck. The first common result obtained from these methods was, on the one hand, the rehabilitation of psychological thinking on the psychopathology of schizophrenia; this was a cautious rejection of Jasper's psychology of meaning, along with its inferred theory of incomprehensibility; and, moreover, this was achieved, at least by the above authors, quite independently of psycho-dynamic schools. On the other hand, they also suspended the tradi-tional somatome-postulate and developed a pure psychopathology free from constant reference to the biological cause of illness. Instead of being inferred, either separately or as a whole, from a presumed so-matic impairment, symptoms were deduced and embodied in a kind of mental entity discernible only by the means of psychology, and sub-jected in its origin and manifestation to certain rules. However, this inevitably led to a mistrust of the validity of Kraepelin's dichotomy, furtively reviving the stage concept of unitary psychosis. This is clearly exemplified by Conrad, Janzarik and Weitbrecht.

Those considerations had little impact on practical diagnosis, which invariably continued to use the Kraepelin-Schneider categories. Delu-sional perceptions, hallucinations, etc., continued to be spoken of, with-out being regarded as symptoms in the medical sense or as signs in the terms of K. Schneider, but rather as terminological abbreviations for psychopathological events. Although the Kraepelin-Schneider catego-ries lost their diagnostic weight, they continued to be investigated and efforts of understanding them psychologically continued but to be just beginning with their denomination. A special place is given here to Huber's work. He followed mainly Conrad's second idea and en-deavored to interlock closely pathosomatic findings with basic schizo-phrenic disturbances, aiming at equipositioning the nucleus of schizophrenic illness and organic psychoses.

The existential-anthropological viewpoint, represented by its most eminent authors such as Straus, Von Gebsattel, Zutt, Blankenburg and, of course, the Swiss Binswanger, pursued another goal. The contribu-tion of this research line consists mainly in the radical discarding of the traditional model of disease, as well as—consequently—in the new critical revision of the notion of mental abnormality (reference litera-ture in Glatzel 1973, 1978, 1981). The starting point for describing mental variety is no longer a norm independent of the person under consideration, but rather the individual biography itself, reflecting the meanings of particular experience and behavior. Extensive case studies are designed to elucidate individually specific displacements and distortions of basic anthropological structures.

Originally, the comprehensive structures of the alienated self- and world-concept, such as those of the delusional, are delineated, so that they can be projected upon the sound structure of the being-in-the-world (In-der-Welt-Sein). Thus, the single case analysis is concerned with individually specific aspects of the structure transformation, revealing connections for instance with some biographical determinants, with personal attitudes and expectations as well as with the physiological events of the particular human being. A significant element of this method, also shared by the psychodynamic schools, is the emphasis of the time dimension. Mental life, along with schizophrenic symptoms, is interpreted as a process and not understood as static productions of the sick psyche in terms of the signs of traditional psychopathology. It is also true of anthropologically oriented psychiatry that it preserves the conceptual framework of traditional psychopathology, thus using the traditional language of diagnosis. However, it uses those categories in a new meaning, seeing in them nothing more than some preliminary denominations, their actual content being revealed by means of subtle case analysis alone. The question of causation here too is not considered, i.e., the existential-anthropological approach to schizophrenia also practices a pure psychopathology. In this respect, along with the earlier mentioned unitary-psychological concepts, it is similar to interactional psychopathology (Glatzel 1973, 1978, 1981), which is likewise preoccupied—though not exclusively—with psychoses of the schizophrenia group.

The concept of interactional psychopathology results from the arguments against the premises of a kind of psychopathology considered to be bound to the naturalistic paradigm. On the one hand, it is related to anthropological psychopathology and, on the other, to communicating theoretical standpoints as well as to the interpersonal theories of dynamic psychiatry. The goal of both anthropological and interactional psychopathology is a kind of conflict-oriented research, aimed not so much at verbal statements susceptible to operationalization as at an adequate way of understanding the human being. Unlike anthropological psychopathology, however, interactional psychopathology operates within the field of intersubjective experience, preceding the anthropological categorization since it deals mainly with the discerning of psychopathologically relevant disturbances of relationship rather than with the anthropological method for concluding on anthropological disproportions. Communication theory, psychodynamic psychiatry and interactional psychopathology are related in their common effort to develop a concept of psychopathological relationship implementing certain terms and constructs of a modern interactionism. Unlike theoretical family studies, however, it is not designed to delineate pathogenic communication patterns, forcing one of the partners into abnormal experiences and behavior. Within the framework of interactional psychopathology diagnosticians are not observers judging the relationship between two partners, but someone taking part as if they were participating psychopathologists, analyzing their own perceptions of interactional dissent between the patient and themselves, which form their impressions of mental abnormality. Interactional psychopathology does not compete with the methods mentioned above; instead, it is defined as a precursory way of comprehending mental abnormality, which precedes the interpretation of the impressions in terms of a psychopathological symptom or an anthropological radical.

Communication and family-theory studies on schizophrenia have been slow in gaining consideration in German psychiatry. What those conceptions, represented and complemented in the German-speaking countries by, among others, Richter and Stierlin, have in common is their attempt to infer the manifestation and the appearance of schizophrenic psychoses from some particularities of the relationship and the communication patterns characteristic of the given social context in which the patient is an integral part of the communication-structure—as a rule the family. Psychoanalytically oriented contributions describe the schizophrenic as playing the role of someone upon whom the dominating community members project their suppressed desires and unfulfillable claims or with whose help they are trying to complement or compensate for their own deficiencies and frustrations. The patient becomes a victim with whose help the others stabilize their threatened ego-identity, their deficient ego-strength. Communication-theoretical research, on its part, emphasized the role of the distorted and hypocritical communication patterns, allowing the weaker partner to act and react in the role, i.e., through the symptoms, of a schizophrenic person alone. Here, it is not the dominating partners who ensure their inner stability and relative harmony by projecting and by compelling the other, the weaker, partner to serve the compensation of their deficiencies; from this point of view, it is the community, the framework of relations as a whole, that needs to designate a schizophrenic to prevent its own breakdown, threatened by the pathological structure of communication.

Summarizing the recent stand of the diagnosis of schizophrenia against the background of this outline, one could arrive at the following conclusions:

Formally, the diagnostic criteria of naturalistic origin dating back to the era of Kraepelin and K. Schneider are still valid. The discrimination of the psychoses of the schizophrenia group from those of the affective

type is based invariably on the same traditional symptoms. The implications of diagnosing schizophrenia, however, have been subjected to
a radical change by means of being restricted and broadened at the
same time. The restriction was a natural consequence of a gradual
discarding of one sided medical concepts in psychiatry. The overwhelming majority of authors regard neither the symptom nor the
syndrome as representing a hypothetical biological disease process
notwithstanding the role that is largely ascribed to a pathosomatic
factor in the cluster of causes responsible for inducing a schizophrenic
psychosis. Schizophrenia denotes not only a disease entity, but a pure
psychopathologically founded convention, too. The compelling consequence of the path from nosology to typology was a considerable
diminution of the weight of diagnosing schizophrenia. Establishing
schizophrenia is less important in terms of predicting its etiology and
pathogenesis; it is more relevant in denoting a particular group of
manifestations of mental abnormalities responding probably favorably
to certain therapeutic strategies—both somatic and sociotherapeutic.
The significance of the traditional types of schizophrenia is further
reduced by the established knowledge that at least the course they take
is modifiable by peristaltic factors. Instead, what is of greater interest
is the particular featuring together with the individual determinants,
providing some guidelines for therapeutic intervention.

However, the implications of the diagnosis of schizophrenia have
also been broadened. Renewed cooperation between psychopathology,
psychology and sociology has inevitably led to the insight that schizophrenia is neither an illness of certain parts of the personality nor a
deformation of innate capabilities but rather a peculiar mode of existence, i.e., a global transformation of perception and behavior signalized
by symptoms without being reflected in them. Thus, tracing all particularities of this transformation in every single case becomes the main
task. The idea of a transindividually valid schizophrenia is no longer
tenable. Instead, the individual schizophrenic patient has become the
only subject of investigation. With the abandonment of the naturalistic
paradigm, the nomothetic viewpoint as the main approach to schizophrenia has been replaced by a more idiographic one.

The Affective Psychoses

Conceptual changes in the domain of affective psychoses—for which
K. Schneider coined the term *cyclothymia*—have not been as radical as
those with respect to schizophrenia after Kraepelin. There is overall
agreement on the characteristic symptomatology and on the useless-
ness of attempts to rank the symptoms in this field, as has been done

in the diagnostics of schizophrenia. Likewise, the efforts to distinguish between separate forms of manic and depressive illness have also more or less come to an end with the work of Weitbrecht. Research since Kraepelin and K. Schneider has provided evidence for only three changes to be made in the concept of cyclothymia. The first concerns the unit of cyclothymia, the second the dividing line between psychotic melancholia and psychopathic-neurotic disturbances, and the third deals with the statement reiterated by K. Schneider and his disciples that cyclothymic depression—melancholia—proved to be extraordinarily resistant to environmental insults.

The clinical and genetic unit of Kraepalinian manic-depressive insanity was questioned even in his own day. Discussions first centered on the quest on whether involutional depression should be given a special position. Kleist and Leonhard were the most convinced that grouping together the monopolar depressive and circular courses of illness under the abstract term of manic-depressive disease was no longer justified.

While many German textbooks still present the unrevised notion of the unity of manic-depressive illness, i.e., cyclothymia, postulated chiefly by K. Schneider, a good majority of clinical psychiatrists have discarded Kraepelin's dichotomy. Impressed mainly by the works of Angst and Perris, most clinicians singled out involutional melancholia regarding its clinical and genetic distinctions as firmly established. On the other hand, despite some assertive evidence, there has recently been no uniform answer to the question of whether one should discriminate between cyclic and monopolar depressive courses of illness. The positive answer is supported by investigations on the personality structure of endogenous depressives carried out mainly by Tellenbach and von Zerssen. Accordingly, the characterological traits of "typhus melancholicus" appear to be detectable chiefly in probands with monopolar melancholia, while the features of the "pykniker" described by E. Kretschmer are seen mostly in patients with a circular course of illness. The question of whether those characterological criteria were really suitable for further subdividing manic-depressive illness should be considered still open for discussion, not the least in the light of Matussek's comparative studies of the personality structure of endogenous melancholics and neurotic depressives.

The first impetus to loosening the rigid borders between endogenous and neurotic depressions came from, among others, Weitbrecht (1953). The "endoreactive dysthymia" he conceptualized has no role in today's diagnostic practice; however, it stimulated arguments that by no means are over yet. Starting from a nuclear cyclothymic group, there was the task of setting new boundaries, first to other endogenous psychoses and, second, to those of manifest depressive disorders belonging to the area of neuroses and reactions. Thus, attention was drawn again to those mixed cases (Zwischenfälle), the existence of which was fully acknowledged by K. Schneider on the background of his—still unquestioned—conviction that schizophrenia and cyclothymia would differ only as regards typology, but could not be otherwise differentiated. What is meant is that the bipolar cyclothymias display in their course, along with delusions attributed generally to schizophrenia, perceptual disorders that clinically are hardly distinguishable from episodical schizophrenias. Terms such as "zykloide Psychosen" (cycloid psychoses) as well as such diverse subtypes as "Angst-Glücks-Psychose" (fear-happiness psychosis), "Verwirrheitspsychose" (confusional psychosis), and "Motilitätspsychose" (motility psychosis) began to appear in hospital statistics along with the several forms of the "Emotionspsychosen" (emotional psychoses) of Labhardt. Depending on the author's scientific standpoint, this was either a return to the time before Kraepelin with its diversity of independent endogenous diseases or a revival of the idea of one single endogenous unitary psychosis. Practical diagnosis, however, has not benefited appreciably from the renewed interest in the border area between the cyclothymias and the schizophrenias; only schizoaffective psychosis (Kasanin) has acquired a firm position.

More important than the question of whether to include in diagnostic nomenclature various terms of the past and present denoting this particular psychopathological evidence, however, were the consequences for the notion of endogenous psychoses in general and especially for the schizophrenias of investigations of the "mixed cases." They shattered the dogma of the autonomy of those mental diseases, thus making the de-emphasis of the rigid endogenicity concept more plausible. Results were afforded by the tentative description of separate forms of manifestations of cyclothymic depressions depending on the presumed provoking insult. This is exemplified by the "Erschöpfungsdepression" (exhaustion depression), the "climacteric depression" or the "Pensionierungsbankrott" (retirement bankruptcy). However, the masked depression ("Larvierte Depression") definitely does not belong here, but to the nuclear group of cyclothymic depression, since in this case there are "classical" symptoms of endogenous depression relegated to the background by somatic complaints (Glatzel, 1985).

The transitional zones between cyclothymic depression and neurosis were made the subject of discussion by K. Schneider himself, who described "Hintergrunddepression" (background depression), followed by Weitbrecht with "endoreaktive Dysthimie" (endoreactive dysthymia). Attempts of this kind are basically bound to an old idea raised again recently also by Tellenbach and Janzarik—appearing first in a well-known publication of Reiss. According to it, the various forms of manifestation of affective disorders can be distributed along a spectrum, with the autonomous manic-depressive disorders placed at one end and the personality-bound constitutional affective disturbances at the other. All disease pictures situated along the spectrum can shade imperceptibly into one another.

Diagnosis in the field of cyclothymia, i.e., affective disorders, in German-language literature may be summarized in the main as follows. Schneider's old cyclothymia has shrunk to a nuclear group. It comprises involutional depression, regarded as clinically and genetically independent, as well as the monopolar and cyclic forms of illness, the autonomy of which, although not generally recognized, is stressed by certain authors. The phenomenological connections with the schizophrenia group have become closer—perhaps significant for a development leading from Schneider's de-emphasis of Kraepelin's dichotomy to the concept of unitary psychosis represented by a virtually unlimited number of psychopathologically defined preponderant types. The phenomenological penetration of melancholia into the area of neuroticism necessitated a departure from the conviction that affective disorders had a special environmental stability and autonomy, and stimulated research into the predepressive causative areas of those diseases in terms of delineating particular predispositional traits of personality or describing specific pathogenetic patterns within the environment.

As in schizophrenia, there is a marked trend also in the diagnosis of affective disorders toward replacing the idea of a transindividually uniform illness by the concept of specific expressions of mental abnormality, innate in every individual, with a limited number of phenomenological similarities contrasted with a large number of phenomenologically and etiopathogenetically more significant individual features.

Psychopathic Personality

Discussion in German-speaking psychiatry on the concept and the diagnostic relevance of the term "Psychopathic personality" (psychopathische Persönlichkeiten), and "Psychopath," respectively, have a long and unusually stirring history (summarizing literature, e.g., in Häfner, Kallwas, Tölle, Petrilowitsch). The term is nowadays either completely avoided or replaced by a less offending one. Leonard, for instance, speaks of "accentuated personalities" (akzentuierte Persönlichkeiten), denominating actually any mental disability of psychiatric significance.

Present discussions in German-speaking psychiatry on the problem of psychopathy should be seen against the following background:

K. Schneider's concept of psychopathy was based on three internally consistent premises: the statistical notion of norm, the placing of psychopathy within the systematization of mental illness and, thirdly, the idea of a primarily hereditary-constitutional predisposition toward psychopathic aberration of personality. Schneider's statistical concept of norm was considered not only to be free of value judgment, but also as demanding the linking of the notions of normality to an external, i.e., verifiable, criterion. This is of a special importance here. Freud, on his part, had pointed out what is now self-evident, that "normality" cannot be considered identical to imitative conformity and "averageness." He described normality as a constantly endangered balance between consciousness and repression, as an extremely individual ratio, conceiving it as an attemptable but unreachable goal of perfect stability. In terms of Freud and K. Schneider, mental abnormality acquires the quality of an attribute, a characterological variant, allowing—once established—not only communication with patients but their estimation and perhaps condemnation as well.

The inconvenience of this sort of systematization of the individuals who characterize those concepts of psychopathy was emphatically articulated by the school of existentialism (Daseinsanalyse), which provided the guidelines for Häfner's instructive research on psychopathy. Häfner defined "the fictitious fulfillment within non-authentic existence" as essential to the psychopathic mode of being. Thus, the anthropological-existential viewpoint made the issue of psychopathy accessible to the sociologically trained eyes of scholars otherwise quite remote from Binswanger's reasoning. A keyword within the frame of reference is the concept of the "façade." The gap between actual existential stagnation of some particular modalities of being, innate to the psychopathic constitution, on the one hand, and the lack of fulfillment of false ambitions, on the other, is bridged over, in Häfner's terms, by a fictitious solidity of the façade. "Façade" denotes here a specific mode of "being-together" (Mitsein), allowing the psychopath to maintain no more than insufficient, especially poor, mutuality. The concept of the "façade"-like communication style, a disturbance of the mutuality of expectations, refers to certain characteristics excluding the psychopathic constitution from the traditional norm concepts meant to define any form of deviation either by the standards of a "presumable average" (K. Schneider) or in terms of a relatively successful accord between the incompatible demands on the various personality levels. Conceptualizing psychopathy as a perverted mode of communication, however, means treating this highly disputed "psychopathological establishment" from a sociological standpoint. The "other" person, or the person opposite, no longer acts in the role of the competent observer "diagnosing" a psychopathy from the distance of carefully safeguarded competence. Instead of the role of the erudite interpreter, one now takes over that of the partner engaging in the mode of "being-together" we call psychopathic. Accepting such an attitude means discarding the traditional medical-psychiatric approach. At the same time, it also implies depriving the concept of disorder, which is closely linked to the standards or norm for every curative branch of medical knowledge, of its meaning and applicability. In all psychiatric statements on the subject of the "psychopathic" or "abnormal" personality, talking about abnormality presumes a kind of disturbance in the sense of constraint, loss of liberty, reduction, disharmony, disequilibrium. Such an understanding of mental abnormality was, finally, indispensable for the claims of a post-Kraepelinean psychiatry to competence with regard to the identification, classification, evaluation, and perhaps the care of the psychopathic person. The attempt to reformulate and elaborate the subject of psychopathy in the context of a theory of social interaction, however, renders it impossible to connect abnormality—taken as a specific form of deviance—with destruction, menace, disturbance or disorganization. Deviation, after all, can also support quite effectively a predefined organization.

"Psychopathy" or "psychopathic personality" is thus no longer considered a sum of the dysfunctional, troublesome mental handicaps and displacements. These terms denote, rather, unpredictable behavior that cannot be explained in terms of conventional concepts of norm and disturbance. This behavior can be tested at most for its appropriateness—provided the expectations of those with whom the psychopath is interacting as well as the actual situations are known in advance. Thus, a person acting contrary to norms in a given or possible situation could be designated a psychopath in the sense of Canguilhem, but so could as well the person who is incapable of transgressing the temporary standards of normality. While the attempt to discuss the concept of psychopathy within the context of social interaction is basic to psychiatry, sociologically inspired contributions to the problem of its causation seem to serve no other purpose than as reference to an obviously forgotten tradition of medical psychiatry. The objections to Schneider's postulate of constitutional deficiency were raised earlier in the teachings of so-called anthropological medicine in the early 1920s. Similarly intended sociopsychological investigations designed to elucidate psychopathy caused by specific conditions of socialization need not be reviewed here in detail. Irrespective of their possible significance in overcoming the fatalistic attitude of traditional psychiatry to psychopathy, there was no need to take the roundabout way through sociology to achieve this result. By turning to sociology to elucidate psychopathy, psychiatry turned back to ideas it had largely ignored for years on end during its gradual development as a specific branch of medicine. Brought back to this early stage of thought, however, psychiatry was now able to approach psychopathy from a different viewpoint, considering strictly the findings and theories of the social sciences while outlining its own hypotheses. Classical psychopathology, based in its general part on Dilthey's structural psychology, saw understanding as the most important access to the so-called psychopathological establishments. However, in its treatment of psychopathy by emphasizing the hereditary dispositional component it abandoned just that perspective of an "understanding psychology." This apparent inconsistency may have arisen partly because psychiatry, following its own claims and fulfilling the expectations of criminal justice, had illegitimately usurped a field without having the knowledge or methods to cultivate it. Bound to medical concepts of illness, it may find itself justified in considering mental illness its genuine field of research—justifiably at least insofar as endogenous psychoses have, at long last, been rendered also "somatically determinable."

Even though psychiatry lacked a proper psychology of its own, was not associated with the progress of medical anthropology, and confronted the social sciences with only skeptical ignorance, it nevertheless successfully annexed the "abnormal variants of mental life" (abnorme Spielarten seelischen Lebens—K. Schneider) by pronouncing them manifestations of a constitutional disharmony, analogous to the "inborn error" in modern medicine. Thus, there is no more room for the intuitive apprehension and understanding of such a "per dispositionem" aberrant personality, since a therapeutically inspired attitude of this kind would inevitably crash upon the rocks of characterology. Instead, psychiatry, on the one hand, decided on a concept which separated abnormal personalities from curable patients who demanded therapy and, on the other hand, tried to provide society with clues for a legitimate strategy of controlling dysfunctional persons who are not ill. This standpoint, reflecting the impotence of psychiatry rather than a critical insight, relegates abnormal personality to the preventive perspective of the social sciences. Psychiatry thus implies that it cannot treat psychopathy. Any further discussions of the problem would be worthwhile only if psychiatry accepted that the Social Sciences could contribute to the prevention of psychopathy in terms of the system of psychopathy that psychiatry holds. A way out had to be found from the contradiction of psychiatry regarding psychopaths in sociological terms and trying at the same time to describe them in terms of one or another preponderant theory of personality. This could, in effect, mean nothing more than the suspension of a tradition stretching from Koch to Schneider, and its replacement by the modern social-science theory of deviance, which is critical of the traditional preventive perspective. Only through a decisive change in thinking in this sense, which would mean also a return to some buried reference points of early psychiatric research, could the discussion of the psychopathologically abnormal be linked to a manner of viewing and understanding the mental variance marked quite clearly by Jaspers though later abandoned almost entirely in clinical psychopathology. In their criticism of sociology before World War I, Sutherland, Lemert and other authors of the so-called Chicago School demanded that the standpoint of those subject to investigation be accepted while studying the content, structure and norms of dissocial marginal groups. It is the task of the sociologist to interpret the world as it appears to the person affected. In the case of research on psychopathy, to precede all classifying or typifying of psychopathic personalities by an individually relevant, i.e., behavior-relevant, definition of the situation for every single case. Such a change in viewpoint, looking primarily for the meaning of the actual situation to the psychopathic deviant, is naturally bound to lead to a de-emphasizing of widely used terms such as disturbance, disorganization and dysfunction. But it by no means implies the romanticizing blindness of some of psychiatry's present critics to the subjective suffering of the drop-out from the conventionally defined situation. The psychiatry of psychopathy learned together with sociology, and from the same evidence, that the naturalistic methodology of early sociology could result in hasty, deadlocked findings that would mislead further research. Such a shift to the viewpoint of the deviant personality itself—to the acceptance of the person's own definition of the situation—contradicts the typical aim of traditional psychiatry to reduce the unconventional, i.e., non-conformist and alien to expectation, attitude and patterns of behavior to a single or several characteristic traits or ingredients of the personality (e.g., weak willpower, unsteadiness, lack of self-reliance). It leaves to a special type of investigator, for example, a forensic psychiatrist, devoted to compiling catalogs of features of directly observable and inductively established patterns of behavior, to develop strategies for restricting, labeling or, at least, rejecting people who disturb a particular predetermined organization. However, such an investigator would be bound to impede the élan of research, which seeks to clarify the meaning and the importance of the established deviance. The degree to which traditional teaching about psychopathy drew on early naturalistic sociology shows in its still continuing effort to distill convenient typologies of abnormal personalities, which are designated according to rules and norms that are especially evident and lastingly disturbing when violated.

Instead, much less effort was spent on the task of describing, for example, how juvenile psychopaths spend their day, and how they reason about their deeds and about society. So, not surprisingly, the younger critics of such a notion of psychopathy reversed the lance and declared that the problem is not that of deviant outsiders, typified in one way or another and breaking established rules of behavior, but rather that of their judges who adhere to a predetermined code. Those critics certainly did not consider that what they saw was less a significant psychopathological point of reference than a helpless psychiatry seeking refuge in, and borrowing from, the social sciences. Dealing with the problem was certainly not helped by such a change of roles, the deviant rendered conformist, and the conformist labeled deviant or at most, the understanding that the preventive perspective itself indispensably requires a discussion of the allotment of power within a given society, a problem that for its part definitely and according to everybody exceeds the field of psychiatric competence.

Nevertheless, the exceptional popularity the concept of role-changing has gained in psychiatry—and not only in the context of psychopathy—exemplifies a general trend in certain sociological theories of deviance. It is a question of weakness in the usual understanding of deviance, pointed out already by Durkheim's investigations on suicide, to which the psychiatry of the abnormal personality is bound to be especially susceptible. What is meant is the belief, contradicting reality, that it is possible to draw a sharp line between deviant and the conformist behavior, which gives reason to assume that the group of psychopaths, kept together by the feature of abnormality, is a relatively homogeneous entity whose representatives share more common traits between themselves than with the others—the conformists, the unobtrusively adapted. Speaking of the "group of psychopaths" was made possible only by a reasoning of this kind, estranged from reality and adhering basically to the medical concept of pathology. Accurate studies by Goffman, Becker, Lemert and others have shown, however, that deviance and conformity are not sharply delimited but overlap widely and gradually. Overlapping does not yet mean a gradual transition from the normal to the pathological which psychiatrists have always attempted to convert into a definable border zone by applying an arbitrary external criterion: the so-called statistical norm. Instead, this overlapping implies more. In the first place, it implies that any psychopathic behavior is a highly complex phenomenon consisting of interlocked deviant and conformist aspects, with the borderline between both varying with the question of the particular meaning of the specific behavior. This insight was also available to psychiatry from the social sciences earlier, for example, from Max Weber, who concluded that empirical research on social behavior was possible by understanding its "meaning" alone. Psychiatry could be facilitated in disavowing its futile efforts toward a topological classification of psychopathic structures, first of all by the future critical extension of Weber's concept of social behavior, which accepted that supra-individually valid and autonomously established patterns of meaning are also to be taken into account in the interpretation of the laws of human behavior along with "the subjectively interpretable meaning."

It was mainly with the help of this concept that the social sciences successfully substituted for the concept of pathology (originally inherited from medicine) that of complexity, i.e., diversity, by juxtaposing the convincing alternative of the functional meaning of deviant behavior to the prevalent notion of prevention. This implies in effect that specific nonconformist patterns of behavior, when analyzed in detail, cannot be ascribed to a deformed structure, however well established, but rather that their meaning must be sought, i.e., the functions they fulfill in a given situation. In doing so, however, the emphatic error of modern psychiatric criticism of simply equating the meaning and functionality of a particular behavior must be avoided. Dilthey, who also insisted on the need to understand the seeming meaninglessness of particular life-forms as an impetus to restructuring them within a new framework through an "intellectual process of highest exertion" so as to still be able to grasp the meaning of the whole, likewise did not mean that the conceivable sense is necessarily functional. Meaningful behavior is often rather dysfunctional, irrespective of the perspective of the fortunes of the individual or of society as a whole and its cohesive order. Likewise, behavioral dysfunctionality should not be confused with abnormality, unless a "normal" coping strategy is determined for every imaginable situation from the unlimited number of possible strategies. Dysfunctionality does not mean a psychopathic, or even a disturbed, personality unless a true social phenomenon is misinterpreted because of the characteristics of personality.

Thus, no systematization of abnormal personalities is at all possible; at most there can be a necessarily incomplete enumeration of certain preponderant types. Those catalogues vary with their author's school of thought, in regard to both the number of components and the defining features. Some investigators, such as Huber and Petrilowitsch, in the true tradition of German psychiatry, immutably rely upon the nonsystematic typology of K. Schneider. The fact that Huber's classification, for instance, speaks first of "personalities" and then of "psychopaths" illustrates its, at least, subtle valuative aspect. Its valuative aspect is closely connected to the underlying concept of personality, which is conceived of as something basically predetermined in its defining features. Accordingly, the types of abnormal personalities are the results of depicting the traits and motivations of the personality that are directly accessible to observation, i.e., description. Thus, what those authors mean by "psychopathy" and "abnormal personality" is a statement on phenomenology but not on pathogenesis. The unifying characteristic of the latter group consists in the exaggeration of "normal" traits which obtrusively dominate the picture.

Notwithstanding that this concept of psychopathy can still be found in several German-language textbooks, it can no longer be considered the predominant concept. The influence of psychodynamic thought in all fields of psychiatry has led to the replacement of the originally rather static concept of personality by a dynamic one, and this has resulted in the incorporation of psychopathy largely within the neuroses. This trend is logically reflected in the replacement of the term "psychopath" by "psychopathic development." Consequently, the common features of psychopathy are likewise no longer seen in separate predominant traits but rather in certain innate dynamic patterns expressing themselves in specific faults of attitude. This notion is found especially clear-cut in the psychoanalytic teaching on nuclear neuroses and character neuroses, represented, for instance, by Reich and Schultz-Henke.

Identifying character neurosis becomes meaningful only against the background of a concept of character rooted in psychoanalytical ego-psychology. One could be aware, however, that—just as the Freudian concept of neurosis rendered mental health, i.e., normality, a fictitious ideal unachievable in the individual—no normal character, or normal character-development, can be identified in reality. According to Reich—and Fenichel to some extent—a society that would tolerate normal character development is imaginable, but so far no such utopian social organization has evolved.

The doctrine of character neurosis derived from observations during the psychoanalytic treatment of patients who could not follow, or who followed only reluctantly, the basic requirements of psychoanalysis. Psychoanalysts, convinced that every willing and sensible patient should accept as obviously curative what they demanded of them, were eager to interpret the contradiction or the neglect of basic rules only as a lack of reason or a resistance to be overcome. Fenichel considered that disobeying the basic psychoanalytical rule was a manifestation of "unreasonable behavior," needing analysis. His typology of character neuroses focused on two basic forms of character: the sublimatory type and the reactive type. It implies the objection that the Freudian typology—differentiating between the erotic and narcissistic types—does not comply sufficiently with the dynamic principle of psychoanalysis. Fenichel proposed a subdivision according to the corresponding kind of neurosis, designating the phobic and hysteric type of character along with the obsessive, cycloid and schizoid types. Psychoanalytic treatment, in his view, should aim at loosening up the character neuroses which concealed from the patient his pathological attitudes and impeded the perception of the congenial conflicting energies connected with those attitudes. Old conflicts are to be recovered and remobilized from behind the character-neurotic defence strategies. The personality must be freed from the rigidity that contained the pathogenic energies. Accordingly, character neurosis represents the acquired faulty attitude that has to be removed in order to obtain access to the underlying symptom-neurosis. Hence, all kinds of analysis are to some extent character analyses. Reich obviously shared the same point of view when he said that the neurotic character was congenial to neurosis since it developed upon a neurotic basis. Every single symptom-neurosis was grounded in the neurotic character called into being by the closing of the Oedipal stage. Consequently, there should be no reason for differentiating between actual neurosis and psychoneurosis.

Character neurosis, impeding therapeutic efforts as a sort of armored defence mechanism, submits to the same rules of symptom formation as symptom neurosis. Reich attempted to separate them by pointing out the lack of insight in character neurosis. Only when the neurotic character becomes exacerbated to a symptomatic level does the person feel ill. Moreover, character neurosis is characterized by marked rationalizations that can go as far as making the character neurotic symptom seem a normal personality trait in the long run. Each character, by its primary function, is designed to defend against the outside stimuli and repressed drives. However, the specific shape of the character, its particular mode of armor, depends on several factors. These conditions for character differentiation account for such types of character neuroses as, for instance, the hysterical character, the obsessive, the phallo-narcissistic and the masochistic. According to Reich, the outcome of character formation depends mainly on the following crucial points: the moment of the drive frustration, then the intensity of the frustrating experience and, finally, the sex of the chief frustrating person as well as the contradictions within the frustrating experience itself.

Schultz-Henke's neo-psychoanalysis has contributed to the concept of character neurosis mainly in respect of terminology. Schultz-Henke conceptualized character neurosis as resulting from some inhibited and misguided drives which determine the basic neurotic disturbance of character that generates the neurotic symptoms in situations of "temptation" or "distress." By coining the term "inhibition" Schultz-Henke intended to define more precisely the defence mechanism already described by psychoanalysis. Along with Freud he designated orality, anality and sexuality as the categories of instincts important with regard to neurosis. To those he later added intentionality and urethrality.

Accordingly, character neuroses are generally conceptualized as attitudes and motivations that neither probands nor those around them perceive as mental abnormality. They could be typified as symptomless neurosis or "nuclear neurosis" (Kernneurose) in the terms of J.H. Schultz, only by viewing them as manifestations of faulty attitudes with their own individual history and obeying the same inner law, which psychoanalysis presumes constituted a symptom neurosis.

Obviously, character neuroses can hardly be distinguished from psychopathies of traditional psychiatry, nor can they be separated descriptively. It is a question of the terms that tend to be used in speaking about pre-existing psychopathy or character neurosis, which when analyzed in a certain way can be regarded as a symptom neurosis.

Classifications of abnormal personalities, and psychopathic development, often used today and closely related to psychoanalytical concepts, are presented by Bräutigam, Kisker's group (Bauer et al.) and other authors. Kisker's working group designated two groups of abnormal personalities, including the sensitive, the paranoid and the schizoid into the first group and the hyperthymic, the depressive and cycloid personalities into the second group. The first—abnormal personalities—is characterized mainly by its specific properties of reaction and defence mechanisms such as strong introversion and withdrawal tendencies, and the second—psychopathic development—is based on structural, i.e., constitutional, pre-existing features along with the faulty attitudes that result from them. Hence, the first one seems closely related to the psychoanalytic concept of character neurosis, while the second complies rather with the traditional Scheiderian psychopathies. Bräutigam, on the other hand, differentiated between the body-centered (körperbezogen) asthenic (e.g., depressive, self-conscious and anancastic forms) and the sthenic (e.g., expansive, fanatical, querulous, explosive and aggressive) psychopathic development.

To summarize, there is no evidence in the German-language literature for any fundamental change since the days of K. Schneider in the doctrine on psychopathic personality in its present state with regard to its conceptual denomination. Corresponding to the general modification of the personality concept in the sense of its dynamicization, however, speaking of abnormal personality nowadays no longer implies the notion of a relative prevalence of specific traits of character in the sense of an "accentuated personality" (akzentuierte Persönlichkeit). The term is considered, rather, a predictive statement about certain early acquired habits of reacting which typify probands' relationship to the environment and themselves and which are manifested by a preference for specific psychoanalytically conceptualized defence strategies or defence mechanisms, definable not as symptoms in the proper sense, but rather as particular traits of character.

Neuroses

Unlike other important terms in psychopathology and psychiatry, "neurosis" carries with it etiological implications. Whereas "schizophrenia" or "organic psychosyndrome" implies mainly symptomatology, "neurosis" has etiological implications. Divergent schools of thought agree largely on this. They differ mainly because of different ideas about the mechanism of the origin and about the issue of ubiquity, i.e., the validity of inner neurotical laws that affect both non-neurotic and psychotic mental life.

Dynamic psychology sees neurotic symptoms as representing a compromise between a desire and the defence mechanisms needed to protect against the incompatibility of that desire with the self-image and the expectations of significant others. They are thus the symbolic expression of mental conflict.

Traditional psychiatry understood neurosis generally in the sense of K. Schneider, i.e., as an abnormal reaction to experience, with its particular coloring strictly limited to the individual—thus precluding any deductions about more generally valid modes of functioning and malfunctioning of the "mental apparatus." K. Schneider called the psychology of neuroses the psychology of the human heart itself. Dynamic schools, on their part, answered by juxtaposing the doctrine of symbolism: the neurotic symptom representing a symbol of determining significance (for details on the concepts of symbol see, for example, Freud, Jones and Lorenzer).

According to dynamic psychology, any mental abnormality is, and should be, regarded as neurotic to the extent that the proband's verbal and nonverbal messages can be seen to follow a certain logic beneath their apparent incomprehensibility and contradictions. The concept assumes that any symptom can be detected and decoded, and seen to be an ego-directed processing of unconscious material, i.e., a symbol. Coding, in psychoanalysis, is effected by a few psychodynamic mechanisms which determine all mental life; the therapist must understand them in order to help such patients regain control over their secret desires and motivations. The most complete and largely accepted theory of neuroses is that found in Fenichel's textbook, but it is rarely applied in surveys. Generally, the psychoanalytic teaching on neurosis differentiates between actual neuroses and defence neuroses, i.e., psychoneuroses, and some authors include character neuroses, sexual disorders, the vegetative neuroses and psychosomatic diseases.

Actual neuroses, according to Freud, have three main characteristics: Unlike psychoneuroses, they comprise only recent disturbances of sexual life; they have a somatic etiology; and the symptoms are not a symbolic expression of some coded disturbance, but rather the direct result of sexual dissatisfaction. This Freudian concept of actual neurosis was later modified because of criticism especially of the second and third characteristics. Today, other drives besides the sexual drive are considered to be etiologically important, and the condition is considered an expression of a drive-conflict, its symptoms symbolic in psychoneurosis. Freud himself revised his assertion about somatogenesis at least for anxiety neurosis. Battegay has integrated recent predominant views in German-language literature into the concept that all neuroses, whether actual neuroses or psychoneuroses, are the expression of drive-conflicts; they differ only in the time of onset or the noxae. Where there has been no underlying drive-disturbance since childhood, and the neurosis appearing in adult life is the result of stress, it is actual neurosis (1971). Freud's original concept of actual neurosis is still encountered today, mostly in the explanation of certain psychosomatic disorders. The actual neuroses comprise neurasthenia, anxiety neurosis and hypochondria.

Hereditary influences, according to Freud, are much more important for defence neuroses or psychoneuroses where the cause is less obvious. The concept of defence neurosis was later also enlarged, resulting in today's assumption that other drives, for example, the aggressive drive, can contribute to defence neurosis as well as the sexual drive. Today, the concept of defence neurosis is generally preferred to that of psychoneurosis, because of the observation that mental conflict can be manifested in somatic symptoms, too. When the conflict penetrates into the somatic field, somatic defence processes are released, for example, under cover of an organ neurosis. These were conceptualized by Mitscherlich as a two-phased repression of defence. Defence neuroses include hysteria, phobia and obsessive-compulsive neurosis. In German-language literature, too, the concept of neurosis centred upon the theory of learning is based particularly on Eysenck. He rejected, first of all, the priority of mental complex assumed by psychoanalysis as well as the notion of the secondary role of the symptom. Starting from Watson's conditioning model exemplified by the experiments with little Albert, Eysenck explained why he thought it necessary to consider neurosis a conditioned response. He believed a primarily weak abnormal response was conditioned under the influence of certain situations, and that it could be reinforced later by even unamplified stimuli against the background of some predisposition to particular patterns of behavior. Most important, in his view, are those conditioned responses that generate, for example, the drives of anxiety, hunger and sexuality.

Eysenck tried to specify the concept of neurotic predisposition by means of factor-analytic studies. He defined it as a dimension of personality called neuroticism. His concept of neurosis differs from the psychodynamic one mainly in the new significance he ascribed to the symptom: He did not regard the symptom as a symbol unveiling its own basic meaning when decoded and thus providing an insight into the regulating coding devices. Rather, he considered it an incorrectly learned behavior pattern, inexplicable later except with regard to the underlying predisposition accounting for the occurrence mainly of that particular form of misadaptation. Psychodynamic laws of suprain-dividually demonstrable coding devices are rejected, together with the therapeutic goal of revealing them for the purpose of a causal treat-ment. Far from trying to bridge the undoubted serious differences between the psychodynamic and the learning-theory concept of neuro-sis, it should be emphasized that behavior theory does not take into account (in Scheff's way) modern psychoanalytical literature in claim-ing that psychoanalysis underestimates the individual's social context for the benefit of its special interest in the inner mental processes. The result of the extraordinarily fruitful discussions of the symbol concept in the recent past have refuted these objections.

The concept of neurosis based on learning theory, which considers the symptom identical to the neurosis, excludes all nosology of neu-roses in the narrow sense. There are as many neuroses as there are forms of conditioned maladaptation. Since they all result from the same causative mechanism, the disposition inherent in the personality play-ing merely an unspecific role, the systematics of behavior therapy could be nothing more than a theoretically endless inventory of all imagi-nable forms of human misbehavior.

As regards Eysenck's classification, the reader is referred to the relevant literature.

Wyss, more than any one else, has recently been concerned with developing an anthropological concept of neurosis in the German-lan-guage literature. From this point of view, too, neurosis is conceptual-ized as a conflict between a drive and drive-suppressing factors, neurosis in its proper sense being considered simply an exception among the various possible conflicts and decompensations. Yet, com-munication constraint, communication expansion, and decompensa-tion are integral parts of human existence. And since communication and intersubjectivity necessarily imply conflict, the alternative question "neurotic or normal" becomes irrelevant, since the conflict leads either to communication expansion or to communication constraint. The con-flict, a possible stimulus to the enhancement on the one hand, provokes a decompensation and destruction of "gestalts" on the other.

The anthropological concept of neurosis evolves from an under-standing of the relationship between person, personality and persona as well as from investigations of the malformations and deformations of that relationship.

The anthropological neurosis theory also holds that pertinent psychopathological phenomena must be de-isolated, so that the patient may understand their meaning. The manifestations of illness are to be understood as the expression of the transformed "Gestalt" of the entire human existence. As in the case of the depressions and schizophrenias, the neurosis should also be interpreted in terms of basic disturbances of personal volition, as existential impairments of the growth (Werden) of personality, bearing intelligible patterns of meaning. In neurosis, too, anthropological psychopathology sees an example of a disturbed relationship to future existence (Zukunftsbezug), an impairment of self-realization because of inhibited growth (Werdenshemmung)—in Von Gebsattel's words, by the suspension of gestalt-shaping growth (gestaltschaffendes Werden). In that sense, being neurotic is a kind of missing-your-own-self (Sichverfehlen), a living-beside-yourself (Ansichvorbeileben). Von Gebsattel speaks of the "personal viewpoint" needed to guide the approach to understanding the neurotic. Finally, neurosis always implies the question of the person inasmuch as the neurotic condition deprives the person of his or her self-actualization (Selbstvergegenwärtigung) in Vetter's sense. Although neurotic inhibition of growth is purported to be oriented by the same laws as those that orient the growth of the personality, any neurotic disturbance is bound to be unique, in the same way that the individual personality is unique and incomparable in terms of its particular form of appearance. That is why Von Gebsattel opposes the schematism of the impersonal theories of neuroses, which overlook the fact that individuals fall ill because of their readiness to comply with a schematizing notion such as man; and they also act against all therapeutic support of self-actualization by their dictatorial demands on personal character.

The impersonal coloring of all psychodynamic concepts of neurosis is shown by their attachment to schemes, irrespective of what kind, as well as by the construction of various genetic or phenomenologically descriptive typologies. Accordingly, being neurotic implies a sense of getting lost in impersonal "pre-gestalts" of adhering to forms of self-actualization that impede the development of the unrepeatable individual self into a person and personality. Hence, the basic disturbances in neurosis are the disestablishment of the person (Entthronung der Person) and the process of impersonalization.

These considerations make it virtually impossible to systematize neuroticism from the point of view of anthropological psychopathology. The only possibility would be to designate some distinct forms of neurotic existence which never pertain to inter-individually valid pathogenetic laws. The specific manifestations of the neurotic attitude—depressive, anancastic, etc.—result from biographical-biologically and socially determined patterns expressing the particular inhibitions of personal growth, the unique and incomparable impairments of self-realization.

Organic Mental Disturbances

Bonhoeffer's typifying of organically determined forms of appearance of mental abnormality marks a milestone of scientific development in clinical psychopathology. His doctrine of the exogenous forms of reaction put an end to an obviously futile discussion about the origins of mental disturbances in certain somatic diseases which affect, primarily or secondarily, the brain. The crucial topics of his conceptions are still a point of reference today for every survey in this field. Bonhoeffer postulated, on the one hand, the nonspecifics of noxious agents with regard to the organic, i.e., symptomatic psychoses, thus rejecting the possibility of deducing the noxae from the clinical picture. On the other hand, in his view there is no way of designating the specific psychopathological syndromes that accompany certain organic diseases. Bonhoeffer's second main idea was the conviction that the functional, i.e., endogenous, diseases can be differentiated from those of organic origin by means of a phenomenological description. Clinical psychopathology had to dismiss some postulates from his theory—though without questioning its nucleus: the rule of the nonspecificity of the noxae. It is irrefutable in psychiatry today that each type of mental abnormality can be the result of organic brain damage, and that neither clouded consciousness nor personality destruction and dementia are obligatory signs of symptomatic mental disorders.

As Conrad pointed out in his introductory notes to a widely recognized contribution in a handbook published in 1960, for several decades surveys of symptomatic psychoses have invariably begun with the remark that the very concept was a misconception. This is indisputable. Later, such terms as symptomatic organic, somatically determinable (körperlich begründbar), and exogenous came into use as synonyms, since all differentiation among them is of doubtful value.

To start with, there is no doubt that there are mental disturbances that are connected not only in time with certain manifest somatic diseases affecting the brain, but that present a specific psychopathological coloring as well, and they can therefore be grouped together as a separate type of mental abnormality. By insisting on the clinical heterogeneity of organic, endogenous and neurotic-psychopathic aberrations, i.e., mental disturbances, current psychiatry is confirming Conrad's assertion.

The authors in the tradition of K. Schneider and his psychiatric teaching had good reason to prefer the term "somatically determinable psychoses" (now referred to in English as "psychosis with demonstrable physical basis or somatogenic psychosis"). What they actually sought was an etiological category for the kind of disturbance that could be attributed to a determinable organic lesion with a direct or indirect impact on the brain. Indeed, K. Schneider considered the somatogenic psychoses to be clearly distinguishable in "appearance" from the endogenous ones, though he also emphasized strongly the etiological element in the term. Huber followed K. Schneider's basic tenet and inferred from his own investigations that Schneider's four diagnostic principles in respect of the somatogenic psychoses were still valid as guidelines. Therefore, the phenomenological description is considered to be of undoubted value in their diagnosis, but the final decision rests on etiology. Such an understanding of the exogenous, i.e., symptomatic, psychoses is necessarily linked to the psychiatric-psychopathological belief that the endogenous psychoses differ from the somatogenic primarily in that their causes—presumably biological—have been postulated but not yet established.

This phraseology can be contested only by opposing its underlying and inherent premise—the so-called somatic postulate. However, it should be pointed out that the exogenous psychoses are thus defined etiologically and not symptomatologically, like the endogenous psychoses. The presence of schizophrenia is determined by the amount of demonstrable peculiarities of experience and behavior , i.e., the answer to the question whether a person is schizophrenic depends on the symptoms alone irrespective of their causes. A positive decision is based on establishing the absence of sufficient somatic findings. Yet defining the exogenous psychoses on the basis of symptoms and the endogenous psychoses on psychological grounds raises several difficulties of principle.

Classical German psychopathology, for example, teaches that psychosis should be diagnosed—regardless of type—only by the presence of phenomenological particularities of the presenting picture or of the course of illness or of both. Dysphoria would never be classified as psychotic unless it is associated with a reliably identifiable organic psychosis or accompanied by specific schizophrenic or cyclothymic symptoms. However, the same dysphoria occurring during the confusional convalescence period following brain injury would necessarily be regarded as an organic psychosis, for example, of the so-called "transitional syndrome" (Durchgangsyndrom, Wieck). But not every mental disturbance following a somatic illness would be classified as psychotic; it is up to the examiner to judge whether there is an etiological association.

Therefore, the consequent neuropsychiatric approach identifying the axial symptoms relevant to the differential diagnosis of somatogenic psychoses is only formally consistent with the psychological system in K. Schneider's sense. Fundamental objections to the phenomenological heterogeneity of endogenous and organic mental abnormality show, however, that their concepts of endogenous and organic are basically also arrived at by considering the somatopathological finding, i.e., the somatological frame of reference, in K. Schneider's sense.

Before proceeding to show that this attempt at a definition does not go far enough, I think it may be helpful to review some of the common endeavors for a systematization of the organic, i.e., somatogenic, mental abnormality.

Generally, a distinction is made between acute and chronic somatogenic psychoses. Scheid and Weitbrecht rightly stressed the need to keep apart the paired antonymous terms "reversible/irreversible" and "acute/chronic." The terms "acute" and "chronic" are relevant only to somatopathological changes, and reference to reversibility or irreversibility concerns only the changes of reversal of a given psychopathological syndrome. Thus, acute pneumonia could be accompanied by a reversible delirium, but acute encephalitis could well turn into an irreversible organic psychosyndrome. Conversely, transitory psychotic episodes of clouded consciousness occur in the course of certain chronic infections, for example, tuberculous meningitis, and certain chronic brain diseases lead to irreversible, chronic somatogenic psychoses. Therefore, there is little point in distinguishing between acute and chronic organic disorders unless somatopathological findings are the only basis for the subdivision. After all, certain somatogenic psychoses generally acknowledged as chronic, presenting the so-called axial symptoms of personality destruction and dementia, are seen in acute brain diseases and are often reversible. This means that a classification of somatogenic psychoses should comprise all forms of organically induced mental abnormalities, whether they are considered reversible or irreversible in principle, and whether or not they occur with acute or chronic diseases affecting the brain.

Bonhoeffer, who originated the concept "acute exogenous form of reaction" (akuter exogener Reaktionstyp) and who also emphasized the nonspecifics of the noxae which induce all forms of somatogenic psychoses, was mainly concerned with the psychopathology of acute mental disturbances in certain somatic diseases affecting the brain. Subsequent authors took over the substance of Bonhoeffer's inventory and tried partially to complement it by additional psychopathological evidence so far not classified, and partially to subdivide the complete inventory on the basis of a uniform guideline. Thus, M. Bleuler established his "natural classification of distinct syndromes" of somatogenic mental disturbances, which in Bleuler's systematization are sorted out as separate entities. Conrad in his own classification starts from an idea, at least for the category of the acute disturbances, stated earlier by Ewald, Stertz, Kolle, Specht, Kleist, K. Schneider and many others. It should be agreed, he wrote, that somatogenic psychoses consist of different forms and varieties of the impairment of consciousness. Conrad recognizes the necessity of establishing a concept of consciousness as a premise for defining its impairment as the axial symptom of somatogenic psychoses. Such a definition, however, cannot succeed, and the problem can only be approached by defining it negatively. Starting from unconsciousness, regaining consciousness is characterized by a progressive structuring of the field of consciousness (Bewußtseinsfeld). Finding support in Jackson, Conrad sees in the various forms of somatogenic psychoses different degrees of the destructuring of the field of consciousness. Taking Head's terminology, Conrad describes the somatogenic psychoses as forms of a protopathic transformation of "gestalt" within the field of consciousness which are markedly distinguishable from the "epicritical" field of experience in the state of wakefulness. Protopathic "gestalt"—transformation of the field of consciousness—stipulates a dissolution of the framework of experience, thus liberating properties of "gestalt." Because the somatic noxae continue to be reinforced, a progressive destruction of the patterns of experience occurs, accounting for delusions, hallucinations, confusion and, finally, agony, out of the prodromal signs such as decreasing concentration, irritability, increased activity and emotional disturbances.

Conrad considered his typology as implementing the phase-like sequence of clinical pictures replacing one another.

Adhering to pure phenomenology, the following subdivision seems to apply to the present state of the teaching of organic mental disturbances in the German-language literature. The first group comprises the syndromes characterized by an impairment of consciousness in terms of its clouding. It includes, for instance, the somatogenic psychoses resulting from intoxications or brain injuries, with the clouding of consciousness ranging from light clouding to coma. The second group includes the states of qualitatively changed consciousness. Instead of reduced awareness there is confusion, i.e., a preponderant disintegration of the mental processes. Perception, thinking and emotionality are impaired, resulting in the typical syndromes of simple confusion, oneiroid confusion, delirium and isolated hallucinosis. The third group embraces the pictures of organic change of the personality and dementia of the kind observed after grave cerebral injuries, reduced cerebral blood perfusion or infectious brain processes. Endophorm syndromes, i.e., clinical pictures of somatogenic psychoses equivalent to those of the endogenous diseases, constitute a fourth group. Included also are symptomatic schizophrenias and cyclothymias, which have been seen recently in connection with abuse of drugs, particularly hallucinogens. The fifth group comprises the exogenous psychoses imitating, in their presenting pictures, certain psychopathic constituencies or neurotic symptom patterns. These likewise result from brain trauma or occur in the form of "blunt personality change" in addictions as well as following infectious or acute toxic brain lesions.

Addiction

The abuse of alcohol and drugs is considered to be induced by several factors, including the commercial promotion of some beverages, by associating their consumption with positive social values, and the stimulation by commercial advertising of fictitious needs. Often an important cause of addiction is a conscious effort to achieve the patient-role, justified in many cases by the regular taking of arbitrarily prescribed drugs. In the last instance, along with the actual illness requiring treatment which may result in new addiction, there are the forms of daily mental discomfort which can also provoke a finally uncontrollable drug abuse.

The pathogenesis of addiction is founded on a variety of dispositional and reinforcement elements, of which only hereditary constitutional predisposition and pharmacodynamic factors are mentioned here. The family constellation of early childhood as well as the actual releasing motives are also of great importance in this matter, as are sociocultural influences. Also worth mentioning are those elements of addictive illness that act as stabilizing factors which provide conditioned somatic, mental and social reinforcement.

German-language literature distinguishes between alcohol addiction and addiction.

With regard to alcoholism, Jelinek's subdivision of stages is widely used in the psychiatry of the German-speaking countries to differentiate kinds of alcoholism.

The psychiatry of alcoholism delineates the somatic, mental and social factors of chronic abuse. As to the psychopathological complications, there is a distinction between the actual alcohol psychoses and— as a rule—the degrees of the irreversible personality change determined by the organic brain lesion. Alcohol psychoses include among others the following syndromes: alcohol paranoia (also the form of the delusional mood of being surrounded, in the sense of Biltz (Belagerungserlebnis) or, in most cases, multifactorally determined jealousy); and alcohol hallucinosis along with the Korsakow syndrome and Wernicke's polioencephalitis hemorrhagica superior, belonging likewise to the somatic complications because of the lesions of the eye muscles and ataxia associated with amnesia. Delirium tremens embraces some psychopathological as well as somatopathological findings; it often develops out of a purely vegetative delirium incipient ("Praedelir") not necessarily bound to turn into delirium and provoked in most cases by an involuntary deprivation of drinking. Hallucinosis, on the other hand, not necessarily limited to acoustic misperceptions, occurs during both excessive drinking and alcohol-free periods. It is generally agreed with Benedetti that alcohol hallucinosis that lasts six months usually takes a therapeutically resistant chronic course.

As for addiction to drugs and medicaments, on the one hand, a distinction is made according to the substance taken, and, on the other, special attention is paid to drug addiction in adolescence. Regarding the particular substance, several distinct types of addiction have been described in the German-language literature. Along with growing addiction to tranquilizers, distinctions are also made between the types of addictions to morphine, barbiturates, stimulants, cannabis and hallucinogens. In addition to the well-known data on these, currently and in the context of opiate dependence, the question is discussed whether the response (form of addiction) of the nerve cell is changed under the influence of the poison, and whether the interaction between the nerve cell and the drug alters that response by increasing the activity of the adenylanclase system. It is not clear whether, in the development of morphine dependence, changes in the endorphine metabolism play a role.

The growing number of adolescent drug dependents has not only stimulated intensive efforts at treatment and prevention, but also drawn attention to a particular manifestation of prolonged drug abuse characteristic of young people. It is a case of psychosocial disintegration that could be designated as a "drug-induced syndrome of lack of motivation" (Glatzel).

Gerontopsychiatry

The psychiatric illnesses of old age are generally subdivided according to three main aspects: the disturbances directly bound to the somatic and mental qualities of the last third of a person's lifetime; those with a declining morbidity rate in that age group; and the group of the well-known psychiatric illnesses, showing a relatively typical symptomatological coloring in old age.

The occurrence of the specific mental disturbances of old age is caused by several factors simultaneously. The probable individual life-span is predetermined by certain genetic influences. In many, but not all, cases of mental disturbances of the aged, cerebral lesions play an important role, their effect depending on various peristaltic factors—somatic or psychosocial. It was these factors that allowed Weitbrecht to conclude as early as 1962 that dementia could no longer be considered to be ultimately irreversible. Finally, there are also some general somatic factors, i.e., somatic illnesses, which affect the brain secondarily; psychogenic social factors; and those that typify the decisive qualities of the so-called premorbid personality. It is virtually impossible to compile an inventory of the mental diseases of old age in all their forms of presentation. Only some overlapping preponderant types can be pointed out. Thus, there is the type with predominant cerebral destruction characterized by rigidity, impoverishment, and monotony combined with a tendency to a general flattering of the personality. Those pictures normally pertain to an erosive chronic course. Another type is dominated by anxiety, self-depreciation and vulnerability resulting in a good many cases in a paranoid attitude. In the third type, the general trend toward somatizing, so typical of old age, leads to hypochondriacal reactions and developments which take occasionally grotesque features. Finally, a fourth type is characterized by emotional alterations and a tendency toward neurotic defensive or regressive attitudes.

The organically based psychoses of old age—in the narrow sense—have been subdivided by Lauter (1972) into five independent forms of illness. To Alzheimer's disease he adds senile dementia and the previously separated presbyophrenia to the group of the Alzheimer-type dementias. Further differentiation, either neuropathological or clinical, would not be justifiable. Vascular dementias caused by reduced cerebral blood-flow due to atheromatosis of brain vessels may appear at the same time as senile dementia, but a pathogenetic connection between these two forms of illness is considered impossible. Along with these atrophic processes of known origin there is an extensive group of other cerebroatrophic syndromes resulting from various pathogenetic insults such as infections, toxic and vascular processes, and trauma. The psychoses of the acute exogenous type of reaction specific in causation and appearing in the form of Bonhoeffer's predilection types make up a fourth group. Finally, Pick's disease and Jacob-Creutzfeld's disease are thought to belong to the presenile psychoses. This classification, with its incompatible usage of etiopathogenetic and symptomatological criteria at the same time, is certainly not satisfactory. Yet it is widely applied today in psychiatry in the German-speaking countries.

A number of psychiatric pictures of illness pertaining to any age group are manifested in old age with a relatively specific symptomatological coloring. Psychopathic personality disturbances show more often traits of passivity to the extent of total neglect. Hyperthymic dispositions are either encountered frequently as simple euphoria or they favor development of sexual perversions of importance to forensic psychiatry. Also, alcoholism in old age can be determined by, among other factors, similar psychopathic disturbances. The neuroses of the aged, rooted deeply in the fears of imminent loneliness and the ultimate end, are mostly colored by anxiety or bear hypochondriacal shading owing to the specific trend at that age toward somatization. The depressions of old age or the late cyclothymias, as the case may be, mostly display a mixture of paranoid traits based on anxious hypochondria, combined occasionally with expansive delusions. Just as in the case of the manias of old age, they tend to take a chronic course, developing disturbances of self-estimation which are present also in the intervals between the manic phases. It is characteristic of schizophrenias that the phenomenological boundary between the endogenous and exogenous pictures of illness is blurred, as is that between endogenous and reactive disorders. Furthermore, late schizophrenias are far more symptomatically poor than those of a younger age. Thus, circumscribed delusions are fabulated and symptoms are occasionally reduced to an isolated acoustic hallucinosis. Catatonic schizophrenias are extremely rare at this stage of life. Somatic delusions of influence often bearing a sexual content also play a special role. The organic admixture occasionally accounts for the unusually clear perceptive disorders. The tendency toward a blurring of the boundary between endogenous and reactive pictures of illness is the reason for the description in recent years of a great number of separate discourse types in late schizophrenia. Concepts of the type of "involutional paranoia" and "involutional paraphrenia" are obsolete nowadays; they are considered to be stages of a relatively unitary type of illness—late schizophrenia. Occasionally, a transition occurs from late schizophrenia to a manic-depressive illness, and this has lately led to the revival of the notion of unitary psychosis. Huber's school has pointed out that those late schizophrenias whose symptoms are reduced entirely to qualitatively abnormal body sensations or to noncharacteristic pictures are hardly distinguishable from purely organic syndromes.

Child and Adolescent Psychiatry

The classification of child and adolescent psychiatry does not differ in principle from that of adult psychiatry; that is, the conclusions arrived at in the previous chapters regarding the issues of endogenous psychoses, organic psychoses, neuroses and personality developments are basically valid in this field, too—only the accents of diagnosis are placed differently. The endogenous psychoses are of relatively little importance, whereas the phasic disturbances of development play a greater role. These comprise the psychopathic developments including psychological hospitalism, dissocial behavior and vagrancy, as well as the psychogenous disorders with predominantly somatic symptoms. The crises of puberty and adolescence occupy a large space, especially identity crises and disturbances of psychosexual development, along with incipient sexual neuroses. The same applies to disturbances of the intellect, their variety being attributed to the great number of metabolically determined psychosyndromes. The syndromes of autism are described as subordinate to the endogenous psychoses, playing, as has already been mentioned, a relatively minor part, though clearly differentiated from them. The classification of child and adolescent psychiatry is generally characterized by the fact that it includes most forms of illness distinguishable in adulthood, yet bearing the particularities in presentation and frequency typical of the specific age, which account for their different positioning.

References

Angst, J. Zur Ätiologie und Nosologie endogener depressiver Psychosen. Berlin-Heidelberg-New York 1966.

Binswanger, L. Schizophrenie. Pfullingen 1957.

Blankenburg, W. Der Verlust der natürlichen Selbstverständlichkeit. Ein Beitrag zur Psychopathologie symptomarmer Schizophrenien. Stuttgart 1971.

Bleuler, E. Dementia praecox oder Gruppe der Schizophrenien. Leipzig und Wien 1911.

Bräutigam, W. Reaktionen, Neurosen, Psychopathien. Stuttgart 1968

Conrad, K. Die symptomatischen Psychosen. In: H.W. Gruhle, R. Jung, W. Mayer-Gross und M. Müller (Hrsg): Psychiatrie der Gegenwart Band II. Berlin-Göttingen-Heidelberg 1960.

Conrad, K. Die beginnende Schizophrenie. Stuttgart 1958.

Fenichel, O. Psychoanalytische Neurosenlehre. Bd. 1–3. Olten 1977.

Gebsattel, V.E.V. Prolegomena einer medizinischen Anthropologie. Berlin-Göttingen-Heidelberg 1954.

Glatzel, J. Endogene Depressionen. Zur Psychopathologie, Klinik und Therapie zyklothymer Verstimmungen. Stuttgart 1973, 2. Aufl. 1985, 1. Span. Aufl. 1986.

Glatzel, J. Allgemeine Psychopathologie. Stuttgart 1978.

Glatzel, J. Spezielle Psychopathologie. Stuttgart 1981.

Gruhle, H.W. Allgemeine Symptomatologie (der Schizophrenien). In: O. Bumke (Hrsg): Handbuch der Geisteskrankheiten Band IX, Spezieller Teil V. Berlin 1932.

Häfner, H. Psychopathen. Berlin-Göttingen-Heidelberg 1961.

Harbauer, H., Lempp G., Nissen und Strunk, P. Lehrbuch der speziellen Kinder- und Jugendpsychiatrie. 4. Auflage, Berlin-Heidelberg-New York 1980

Huber, G. Psychiatrie. 2. Auflage, Stuttgart 1977.

Janzarik, W. Dynamische Grundkonstellationen in endogenen Psychose. Berlin-Göttingen-Heidelberg 1959.

Janzarik, W. Schizophrene Verläufe. Eine strukturdynamische Interpretation. Berlin-Heidelberg-New York 1968.

Jaspers, K. Allgemeine Psychopathologie. 8. unveränderte Auflage. Berlin-Heidelberg-New York 1965.

Kisker, K.P. Der Erlebniswandel des Schizophrenen. Ein psychopathologischer Beitrag zur Psychonomie schizophrener Grundsituationen. Berlin-Göttingen-Heidelberg 1960.

Kisker, K.P., Lauter, H., Mayer, J.E., Müller, C., Strömgren, E. (Hrsg.): Psychiatrie der Gegenwart, Bd. 1–9. Berlin-Heidelberg-New York-London-Paris-Tokyo 1986ff.

Kraepelin, E. Psychiatrie. Ein Lehrbuch für Studierende und Ärzte. Band I und II. 6. Auflage. Leipzig 1899.

Lauter, H. Organisch bedingte Alterspsychosen. In: Kisker, K.P., Meyer, J.E., Müller, M. und Strömgren, E. (Hrsg.): Psychiatrie der Gegenwart Band II, Teil 2, 2. Auflage. Berlin-Heidelberg-New York 1972.

Leonhard, K. Aufteilung der endogenen Psychosen. 2 Auflage. Berlin 1959.

Matussek, P. Untersuchungen über die Wahnwahrnehmung. Erste Mitteilung. Arch. Psychiat. Nervenkr. 189, 279 (1952);
Zweite Mitteilung. Schweiz. Arch. Neurol. Psychiat. 71, 189 (1953).

Reich, W. Charakteranalyse. Köln-Berlin 1970.

Richter, H. E., Strotzka, H. und Willi, J. (Hrsg): Familie und seelische Krankheit. Eine neue Perspektive der psychologischen Medizin und der Sozialtherapie. Reinbek bei Hamburg 1976.

Schneider, K. Klinische Psychopathologie. 8. Auflage. Stuttgart 1967.

Stierlin, H. Von der Psychoanalyse zur Familientherapie. Stuttgart 1975.

Tellenbach, H. Melancholie. Problemgeschichte, Endogenität, Typologie, Pathogenese, Klinik, 3. Auflage, Berlin-Heidelberg-New York 1976.

Weitbreche, H. J. Neue Probleme bei cudogenen Psychosen. Nervenarzt 24, 187 (1953).

Weitbrecht, H.J. und Glatzel, J. Psychiatrie im Grundriß, 4. Auflage. Berlin-Heidelberg-New York 1979.

4

The Contemporary American Scene: Diagnosis and Classification of Mental Disorders, Alcoholism and Drug Abuse

Gerald L. Klerman*

I. Introduction: Psychopathology Revitalized

This paper describes the current American psychiatric scene with regard to the diagnosis and classification of mental disorders, including alcoholism and drug abuse.

The Renaissance of Interest in Psychopathology in the 1970s

During the 1970s, American psychiatry experienced a major revival of interest in and attention to issues concerning psychopathology, diagnosis and nosology classification, culminating in the publication of the *Diagnostic and Statistical Manual III* and *III-R* (DSM-III, DSM-III-R) by the American Psychiatric Association (APA, 1980, 1987). Interest in psychopathology has continued through the 1980s.

Because mental disorders are multiple and their treatments diverse, the need for a highly differentiated diagnostic system becomes more important. As Spitzer (1978), who guided the development of DSM-III, has stated:

> The purpose of a classification of medical disorders is to identify those conditions which, because of their negative consequences implicitly have a call to action to the profession, the person with the condition, and society. The call to

* Professor of Psychiatry and Associate Chairman for Research, Department of Psychiatry, Cornell University Medical College, Payne Whitney Psychiatric Clinic, New York, NY.
This paper was commissioned as part of the WHO-ADAMHA Joint Program on Diagnosis and Classification of Psychiatric Disorders. Supported in part by grants R-01-MH-43044 and U-01-MH-43077 from the National Institute of Mental Health, Alcohol, Drug Abuse and Mental Health Administration, Public Health Service, Department of Health and Human Services, Rockville, Maryland, U.S.A.

action on the part of the medical profession (and its allied professions) is to offer treatment for the condition or a means to prevent its development; or, if knowledge is lacking, to conduct appropriate research.

DSM-III incorporated a number of features derived from recent research and clinical experience, the most significant of which was the development of operational criteria for individual disorders—criteria based mainly on directly observable manifestations of psychopathology. Except for the organic conditions, these criteria are generally free of etiological assumptions. In addition, more refined definitions of psychiatric syndromes and delineation of subgroups within the syndromes have also been incorporated.

The renaissance of diagnostic and nosological activity in the United States was accompanied by a division over the balance of scientific and humanistic aspects—a dilemma that exists for all medicine: while the unit of scientific interest is the disorder (or illness), the unit of clinical practice is the individual patient. Put another way; medicine studies diseases, but treats patients (Klerman, 1977; Illich, 1976).

This tension has contributed to continuing controversy and criticism of psychiatric diagnosis. Practitioners have complained that existing classifications hinder clinical practice in at least two ways. First, diagnostic categories are inadequate for understanding the complexity of individual patients and for clinical decision making. For example, it is argued that in evaluating the need to hospitalize suicidal patients, in addition to knowing whether or not the patient is depressed or psychotic, it is also necessary to assess personality aspects, such as the patient's impulsivity or degree of self control, as well as to have an adequate understanding of that patient's life circumstances, particularly current stresses, family and income, and social supports. Second, clinicians have claimed that assigning patients to categories contributes to depersonalization and deindividualization of the doctor-patient relationship.

In response to these criticisms, the DSM-III and the DSM-III-R adopted a multiaxial system. This five-part system consists of

— clinical psychiatric syndromes entailing aspects and symptoms of chronicity and periodicity (Axis I);

— personality disorders of adults and development disorders of children and adolescents (Axis II);

— medical illness (Axis III);

— psychosocial stressors (Axis IV);

— and level of adaptive functioning (Axis V).

The first three Axes utilize categorical judgments, while the last two utilize dimensional rating (Mezzich, 1980).

The DSM-III has generated controversy both within the United States and between U.S. psychiatrists and those from other countries, many of whom follow the World Health Organization International Classification of Diseases (WHO-ICD; WHO, 1980; Skodal, 1982).

Purpose of This Paper

This paper examines the diversity of the contemporary American psychiatric scene against a background of some of the major forces—historical, social and scientific—that have shaped its activities, formed its theories and provided impetus for research and clinical advances. This examination begins with a conceptual perspective from which to view the diversity that characterizes U.S. psychiatry (Section II), followed by an overview of the historical contexts from which multiple schools of psychiatry emerged (Section III); post-World War II developments and advances leading to current emphases on empirical psychiatry are described. Section IV presents the origins, tenets and proponents of the major contemporary schools of American psychiatry, focusing particularly on their views of diagnostic and nosologic efforts. Section V addresses the approaches of the contemporary schools to selected mental disorders, with primary emphasis on research efforts. Section VI concludes with identification of future trends.

II. The Diversity of American Psychiatry

Early in the history of psychiatry in the United States, different emphases emerged for the study and treatment of mental disorders; the biological organism, mental processes (conscious and unconscious), the societal and institutional setting for care and socially adaptive behavior. While the dominance of these emphases has fluctuated at different times, they have provided the basis for the growth of multiple, competing schools, each of which, in turn, has developed its own theoretical, research, clinical and treatment framework.

It is important to recognize that, in the United States at the present time, no school is dominant. Currently, the American psychiatric profession has multiple scientific sources that draw on specialized knowledge within its own broad sphere, ranging from psychoanalysis to psychobiology, as well as on related disciplines of neurobiology, psychology and epidemiology. The diversity characterizing the American professional scene is manifested in considerable ferment and rivalry among the alternative schools. The extent of this diversity has been described by Armor and Klerman (1968), Havens (1973) and Lazare (1979).

Observers of the American scene have cataloged the schools in various ways. In their influential study of social class and mental illness, Hollingshead and Redlich (1958) divided the practitioner community in New Haven into two groups which they referred to as "Analytic and Psychological" (A-P) and "Directive and Organic" (D-O); subsequent researchers employed other groupings. In the early 1960s, Strauss and associates in Chicago (Strauss et al., 1964), using sociological survey methods, and Armor and Klerman (1968), studying a nationwide sample of psychiatrists working in hospitals, identified three psychiatric schools: a biological (or organic) school, a psychological/psychodynamic school and an emerging social/psychiatric school.

Table 1 identifies the five schools most relevant, in this author's view, to the current American psychiatric research scene in regard to diagnosis and classification issues.

Table 1. Contemporary American schools of psychiatry.

—BIOLOGICAL
—PSYCHOANALYTIC
—SOCIAL
—INTERPERSONAL
—BEHAVIORAL

Observers of the American scene will note that a number of influential groups of mental health practitioners are not represented here. For example, the existential school, identified and described by Havens (1973), while influencing many modern philosophers and writers by extending tenets of existential philosophy and literature into therapeutic theory, has had relatively little impact on psychiatric research or practice. Similarly, new forms of psychotherapy, such as Gestalt therapy, humanistic psychology and transactional analysis, that have proliferated in the last decades, particularly among nonmedical practitioners, have often been critical of the psychiatric "medical model" and modes of diagnosis and classification.

The community mental health movement also does not appear here as a separate school; rather, it is regarded as an application of social psychiatry. While it has effected major changes in the delivery of mental health services, its adherents have tended to ignore issues of diagnosis and classification in both their writings and clinical practice. The theoreticians and practitioners of community mental health have been, in fact, at times critical of the medical model and have often been allied on an antidiagnostic position with the antipsychiatry movement.

Ideological Aspects of Schools of Psychiatry

Reference to "schools" of psychiatry in the United States focuses on internal divisions reflecting the different beliefs and cognitive views and practices within the profession. However, it is readily apparent that the ideas and views of these various "schools" are strongly held by their proponents, so much so that discussion of scientific and professional issues among psychiatrists is often attended by dispute, dissension and acrimony. The sociological concept of ideology is useful to describe the complexity of the American psychiatric scene more specifically.

Although most prominently explored and applied in the fields of social, economic and especially political theory (Mannheim, 1936), the concept of ideology has been useful in understanding the processes of cohesion and fragmentation in professions (Strauss et al., 1964; Armor & Klerman, 1968). In the field of psychiatry, a professional ideology may be said to consist of four components: cognitive, descriptive or normative, emotive, and social and affiliative.

Psychiatric schools often become "movements," involving not only the members of the profession, but intellectuals, journalists, legislators and others outside the profession allied with a school's particular views. Thus, we identify a "psychoanalytic movement" or a "community mental health movement," whereas, in other branches of medicine we would seldom, if ever, refer to a "surgical movement" or an "epidemiological movement."

The schools of American psychiatry have differed strongly as to their concepts of mental illness as well as to specific aspects of diagnostic reliability, validity and appropriateness. The differences among the schools also extend to social and ethical issues. Some schools, for example, regard diagnostic efforts as depersonalizing and antitherapeutic and, at times, politically repressive. The force of these ideological elements has often influenced efforts at revision of diagnostic nomenclatures, as witnessed by some of the debates and controversies attendant upon the creation and promulgation of DSM-III and DSM-III-R. My conclusion is that contemporary psychiatry in the United States involves multiple, competing paradigms. It may be that one paradigm will emerge as dominant in the future.

III. The Historical Background

Since its inception and particularly after World War II, multiple schools have developed. This section describes briefly the historical and social forces leading to the differentiation of competing schools after World War II.

The 18th and 19th Centuries

As Foucault (1965) pointed out, the conception of mental disturbances as "illness" was a creation of Enlightenment thinking of the late 18th century. It is not that insane persons or public institutions for their care did not exist before this time; rather, the needs of the mentally ill had been seen until this time as the sole responsibility of law-enforcement agencies or of the church—not of medical specialists and public health administrators. This movement parallels the birth of psychiatry under the leadership of Pinel, who became the first *medical* superintendent of Salpetriere. Salpetriere—involved in the production of saltpeter in the 17th century—was converted first into a hospital for indigents and a few years later into an asylum for madwomen. After a century under political supervision, Pinel, in 1795, unchained the insane and treated them as mentally ill—not as "animals."

The notion of "medical illness" was part of the rational, naturalistic approach to human behavior of Enlightenment thinking. Thus, at the beginning of the American Republic, treatment of the mentally ill was optimistic, reflecting the confidence of the new nation, particularly embodied in the important influence of Benjamin Rush, a signer of the Declaration of Independence and the first American physician to write about mental illness (Musto, 1973).

Psychiatry became a medical specialty in the U.S. in the 1840s with the creation of the Association of Medical Superintendents of Institutions for the Mentally Ill. The dominant approach held by these medical superintendents was known as "moral treatment" (Bockoven, 1963; Rothman, 1971; Grob, 1973). Modeled on the innovative efforts of Pinel in Paris, France, and the Duke of York in England, moral treatment was based on the humanitarian values of the Enlightenment, with emphasis on work and planned activities for patients in a restful, respectful and properly administered environment. The moral treatment of the 19th century provided an antecedent for the mental hygiene movement of the early 20th century and the community mental health movement of the 1960s.

Moral treatment was based on a social approach to treatment of mental illness, legitimizing the authority of the medical superintendent to structure that "moral" environment. In the 1950s, this focus on the hospital environment was evident in the treatment approach known as the "milieu therapy." During both historical periods—the "moral treatment" era of the mid-19th century and the "milieu therapy" era of the 1950s—the attempt was to create an institutional environment that could support and encourage the rationality of patients and their inherent capacity to recover.

In the second half of the 19th century, the moral treatment movement declined in vigor and fell into disrepute. Mental hospitals became overcrowded and increasingly custodial. Various explanations have been given for these changes. Bockoven (1963) attributes much of the decline to the adverse consequences of increasing numbers of Irish, Italian and German immigrants, who overwhelmed and overtaxed public agencies, and the concomitant antipathy of the dominant population to expend monies for services to these "alien" populations. Rothman (1971) also notes the change in demographic character of the patients for which moral treatment had originally been intended. In addition to large immigrant populations, ever-increasing numbers of asylum patients were chronically medically ill and senile, which heightened the tendency toward custodial rather than therapeutic efforts.

The decline in moral treatment was associated with growth of biological theories. Social Darwinism flourished, mental illness was regarded as the inevitable result of "degenerative" process—a view that led to pessimism among professionals, justified "benign" neglect, and shifted emphasis from the therapeutic potential of hospitals to custodialism. In scientific areas, social Darwinism led to a strong interest in the new advances in biology. Activities in bacteriology and pathology derived from French and German laboratories were increasing. These new fields did not, however, have full impact on American psychiatry until after the reforms of American medical schools brought about after the Flexner Report in the early 20th century. At the end of the 19th century, the intellectual and scientific stature of American psychiatry had seriously declined. Its intellectual impoverishment and low professional self-esteem during this period have been described by Hale (1971), Rothman (1980) and other historians.

Until the early part of the 20th century, psychiatry in America, as in most of Western Europe and North America, was almost exclusively practiced in hospital settings. Only a very small number of psychiatrists were in private practice, although many neurologists and other physicians saw psychiatrically ill patients in their office practice. The main concern of psychiatrists was with those disorders that today would be diagnosed as psychotic. Description of various forms of psychoses by Pinel and Esquirol in France and by the German clinicians were readily accepted by Americans. A number of contributions in diagnosis and classification were made in the United States during the latter part of the nineteenth century. These included:

1) *The separation of idiocy from insanity.* This classification may seem self-evident when viewed from the vantage point of the latter part of the 20th century, but this distinction only slowly emerged in the mid-19th century. It was incorporated in the U.S. 1870 census, which counted cases of both "idiocy" and "insanity." This important epidemiological distinction was based on clinical observations that manifestations of idiocy became apparent soon after birth and in early development, whereas insanity occurred in adulthood after apparently normal development during childhood and adolescence.

2) *Awareness of the relationship between life circumstances and mental illness.* The frequency of "nostalgia" as a medical diagnosis was commented upon during the Civil War by many physicians in the Union Army, who observed the symptoms of sadness and grief of young soldiers separated from their homes and families.

3) *Description of the new diagnostic category of "neurasthenia."* Referring to this condition as a disease of American civilization, Beard (1880) described what he believed to be an epidemic of fatigue and weakness, brought about by a rapid urbanization that was "exhausting the nervous system" and causing "weak nerves." A uniquely American categorization, Beard's concept of neurasthenia was popular and provided an apparent neurologic explanation for many bodily and psychological complaints. This theory underlay the work of the neurologist, S. Weir Mitchell (1894), who proposed the therapeutic "rest cure" in which the patient was removed from the family, usually to an isolated rural setting, where rest and rich foods were prescribed and justified by the need to replenish a "weak" nervous system. Implicit in this diagnosis and therapy was a notion that cities and civilization were morally corrupting and causative of mental illness, in contrast to the rural countryside, which was viewed as healthful, refreshing and morally pure. This view became a widespread theme in late 19th-century American writing.

4) *Increased concern about the health hazards of alcohol.* This occurred during the second half of the 19th century consequent to the increase in alcohol consumption. The temperance movement drew public attention to the health consequences of excessive alcohol consumption, leading eventually to enactment of Prohibition laws in 1919.

5) *Identification of drugs leading to addiction.* Morphine derived from opium had come into medical use during the Civil War after the development of the hypodermic syringe and was widely used in

medical practice in the latter half of the 19th century. Musto (1973) has estimated that about five percent of the American population, mostly female, was addicted to opiates during this time. The ongoing effect of morphine addiction upon family life is dramatically depicted in Eugene O'Neill's powerful *Long Day's Journey into Night*, in which the mother's readdiction precipitates a family crisis.

The Beginning of the 20th Century

Most observers of the history of American psychiatry are in agreement that the field reached a low point at the end of the 19th century. The optimism of the moral treatment movement had given way to social Darwinism and custodial practices. In addition, very little research was being conducted, and practitioners attracted to psychiatry seemed to many observers to be of lesser quality than in other fields of medicine.

Some of the most telling aspects of this decline were captured by the neurologist S. Weir Mitchell's lecture to the medical superintendents at their 50th annual meeting in 1894 (Rothman, 1980). An avowed critic of the asylums, he viewed the institutions to be failures as custodial, rehabilitative or teaching settings. Institutions that provided only custodial care could not further the scientific progress of the psychiatry profession: "Where," Mitchell asked, "are your annual reports of scientific study, of the psychology and pathology of your patients? . . . Want of competent original work is to my mind the worst symptom of torpor the asylums now present." He told his audience that so long as "you shall conduct a huge boarding house . . . what has been called a monastery of the mind, you will be unable to move with the growth of medicine, and to study your cases, or add anything of value to our store of knowledge." Even the purist custodial aspect of their jobs was in question: "I have seen hospitals that smelled and looked like second-class lodging houses, and have found their managers serenely contented. You have too long maintained the fiction that there is some mysterious therapeutic influence to be found behind your walls and locked doors. We hold the reverse opinion and think your hospitals are never to be used save as a last resort . . . I think asylum life is deadly to the insane."

Psychiatry as a profession began to change in the decade prior to World War I. It is probably no accident that these professional changes coincided with the emergence of the Progressive movement in American political and cultural life. There seems to be a close historical correlation between periods of improved economic well-being, general intellectual and social ferment, and progressive political movements, on the one hand, and reform in mental health investigators and practices and new ideas in psychiatric professional activities on the other. This pattern was clearly evident in the decade before World War I, when teaching and research activities developed in the new "psychopathic hospitals" in Boston, Baltimore, Ann Arbor and elsewhere. This was also the period during which psychoanalysis had its first impact upon American psychiatric and intellectual thinking after the 1909 visit of Freud and Jung to Massachusetts and other Northeastern states.

The Influence of Adolf Meyer

The influence of Adolf Meyer on 20th-century American psychiatry has been profound and paradoxical (Klerman, 1979). German speaking, educated in Switzerland, France and England, and trained as a pathologist, Meyer was part of a small group that introduced the new European techniques of neuropathology to America. He also helped introduce Kraepelin's concept of dementia praecox to the U.S. academic psychiatric community. Yet, once in the United States, he was strongly influenced by American pragmatism, social psychology and mental hygiene.

Between the time of his arrival in the United States in 1892 as pathologist at the Kankakee State Hospital in Illinois and 1913, when he was appointed director of the Henry Phipps Clinic at Johns Hopkins, Meyer rose to a position of major leadership in American psychiatry. During these decades, Meyer absorbed the ideas of William James, founder of the first American school of philosophy, the social psychology of G.H. Mead and C.H. Cooley at Chicago, and the new psychotherapy of Morton Prince at Harvard. He wrote his comprehensive and scholarly criticism of Kraepelin's concept of dementia praecox, strove to formulate his own dynamic psychology, and broadened the scope of psychiatry to include what he termed "civic medicine" (Rothman, 1980), emphasizing prevention, outreach, and follow-up clinics and programs that anticipated the community mental health movement in the 1960s.

Although Meyer calls his approach "psychobiology," his psychobiological approach is not the same as the current meaning. Today, psychobiology refers to the influence of biological mechanisms, such as chemical and pharmacological processes, upon mental behavior and connotes activities synonymous with biological psychiatry. Rather, Meyer based his ideas on those of Darwin, and he viewed mental illness as an attempt of the individual to adapt to the changing environment, particularly its psychosocial changes. Focusing on patients' lives, objectively and minutely observed and recorded in patients' "life charts," he emphasized maladaptation and habit as being at the core of mental disorder; disease was the "inevitable and natural development from a deterioration of habits due in part, at least, to the clashing of instincts and to progressively faulty modes of meeting difficulties" (Meyer, 1950–1952).

Meyer was the first professor of psychiatry at Johns Hopkins University, which was organized following the reforms recommended by the Flexner Report. The Report emphasized research, professional specialization, scholarship and full-time faculty, and became the model for American medical schools. The few other academic centers of psychiatry that emerged after World War I were most often led by students of Meyer, such as Campbell at Harvard and Diethelm at Cornell. It was through the influence of his students that Meyer's contribution is most lasting; particularly the social psychiatric epidemiology efforts of Lemkau, Rennie, Leighton and others, who amplified Meyer's general approach to identify social factors that generate mental illness and mental retardation in specific communities, were important.

In addition to research in social epidemiology, Meyer influenced the mental hygiene movement, the modification of Freudian psychoanalysis and the emergence of the interpersonal school of psychotherapy. His students dominated the leadership of academic psychiatric centers until well after World War II. Many of the American contributions to psychiatry in the 20th century were the consequence of Meyer's approach, and in many important respects he presaged and effected the diverse directions of the multiple schools on the contemporary American scene.

World War II and Its Consequences

World War II had a major impact upon American psychiatry. The experience of the Selective Service System and of the military led to a greater public awareness of the extent of mental illness and mental retardation. World War II led to increasing optimism concerning the treatment of mental illness.

A group of social scientists within the U.S. Army, led by Samuel Stouffer (1950), developed scales and tests to measure anxiety, satisfaction, fatigue and other psychological states among army personnel. With these methods, they studied the relationship of the stress of combat upon susceptibility to breakdown and psychiatric disease.

After World War II, many of the social scientists involved in military research on stress and performance became active in psychiatric research and continued to study stress and its health consequences. Their focus shifted from the stress of combat and the threat of death to the less dramatic stresses experienced in civilian life, such as poverty, low socioeconomic class, urban anomie and rapid social change (Weissman & Klerman, 1978).

Clinical attention was given to "shell shock" described during World War I and conditions considered "traumatic neuroses." Many forms of psychosomatic disorders were observed, and clinical patterns were found to vary among different armies. During World War I, "soldier's heart" was frequently observed among British troops, and diagnoses of "neurocirculatory asthenia" or anxiety neurosis were common; extensive physiologic and psychological studies of this condition were reported. In contrast, World War II witnessed relatively less cardiovascular disorders, but more reports of gastrointestinal complaints and dissociative states.

Among the most influential American efforts to describe and treat war neuroses were the reports by Grinker and Spiegel in the North African campaign. In their book, *Men under Stress* (1945), they described the use of intravenous amytal to promote therapeutic abreactive reactions. Although these reactions were dramatic, subsequent research by Glass (1955) indicated that this treatment produced only a relatively low rate of return to active duty. Subsequently, the U.S. military modified its psychiatry program, resulting in far less psychiatric disability and morbidity during the Korean and Vietnam Wars.

Brief psychotic states (called "three-day schizophrenia" or "ten-day psychosis") were also reported. These observations seemed to contradict the conventional views of schizophrenia, which emphasized its chronic nature. Although there were many clinical reports of brief transient psychotic states, whose onset seemed to be related to the stress of combat, Glass (1955) demonstrated that while the diagnoses of neuroses fluctuated with combat and occasional transient psychotic episodes undoubtedly occurred, the overall rate of psychoses remained relatively low and stable.

Considerable clinical attention was also given to the forms of personality disorders that rendered individuals unable to cope with military life. Strongly influenced by the psychoanalytic ideas of Karl and William Menninger, precursors of DSM-I were developed in the military psychiatric nomenclatures and in the Veterans Administration classification. They described new conditions, such as "passive-aggressive personality" and "passive-dependent personality."

Post-World War II Developments

The decades following World War II, particularly the 1960s and 1970s, witnessed a proliferation of new theoretical, clinical, and research advances in American psychiatry. These advances included the community mental health center movement and the emergence of behavioral techniques and other new forms of psychotherapy. In addition, the past decade has witnessed a neo-Kraepelinian revival whose adherents consist of a small but energetic group of researchers who began applying statistical and psychometric methods to clinical description and diagnosis, strongly influencing the development of DSM-III.

Community Mental Health Movement

After World War II, mental health issues became matters of national concern. The high rates of mental retardation and emotional and mental disorders reported by Selective Service examinations and the large numbers of psychiatric casualties in the military had attracted public attention during the war. During the post-war period the public was alerted to the mental health needs of the large number of veterans and the alarming increase in patients in mental hospitals. In 1950, one half of all hospital beds in the United States were in mental hospitals.

This public concern resulted in the creation in 1955 by Congress of the Joint Commission on Mental Illness and Health. Its 1961 report, *Action for Mental Health*, called for major reform of patterns of care for the severely mentally ill. The impact of this report was apparent in President Kennedy's 1962 message to Congress, which laid the groundwork for 1963–1965 legislation creating the Federal program of community mental health centers.

During the 1960s and 1970s, Federal leadership and funding contributed to major expansion of community mental health facilities and of professional personnel. Utilization rates increased fourfold in two decades as ever larger segments of the general population sought help from mental health professionals. Considerable debate ensued over the extension of psychiatry into community problems and social issues beyond the traditional scope of psychiatry as a medical specialty concerned with patients with diagnosable disorders.

As in the Jacksonian era of the 19th century and in the Progressive era of the early 20th century, the expansion of psychiatric activities in the United States in the period of the expansion of the welfare state during the 1960s was strongly influenced by national social and political forces. These influences were reflected in differences of theory and practice inside the profession as well as controversy in academic and public policy areas concerning the proper role of mental health in the larger social order.

The Federal community mental health program expanded services to large numbers of persons not previously reached, especially children, the elderly and the poor, while also attempting to initiate prevention and rehabilitation efforts. The rapid growth of these programs generated problems of implementation for the mental health profession and stimulated serious debates concerning evaluation, efficacy and accountability. The movement's achievements were, and continue to be, subject to the vicissitudes of public support and professional commitment. The movement, however, lost most of its programmatic and ideological momentum after the election of Ronald Reagan in 1980.

The Antipsychiatry Movement

During the 1960s and 1970s, an antipsychiatric movement emerged in the United States, with parallel developments in Japan, England, France and Germany. The polemic of Szasz (1961) on the "myth" of mental illness, Laing's (1971) writings rooted in Sartrian existentialism, and Rosenham's study of "pseudopatients" (1973) proved influential in many legal and academic circles.

It is interesting that this movement garnered support in the United States during the decades when psychiatry was pressing far beyond its traditional bounds, especially in community mental health. Although major activity in psychiatry was more directed at this time at programmatic, social and political goals, concern arose over the extension of the mental health profession into social areas where, it was felt, psychiatric expertise could not be justified.

The antipsychiatry writers had a strong influence on the general intellectual thought during the 1960s and 1970s, particularly among sociologists and psychologists, many of whom, known as "labeling theorists," were important teachers in major American universities. Within this framework, mental illness, like other forms of deviance, was viewed as predominantly politically defined and socially reinforced behaviors. Their theories maintained that psychiatric diagnoses of mental illness was a labeling process whereby patients are stigmatized and thereby confirmed in a situation reifying the conditions such labeling was intended to diminish. Further, they held that the stigma separating the mentally ill from the larger population was a form of social control, and that mental health professionals were in danger of becoming instruments of social control rather than advocates of patients' needs (Lemert, 1972; Scheff, 1966, 1975).

The controversies over labeling theory stimulated research on the adverse social and legal consequences of psychiatric practices. Their views strongly influenced many lawyers trained during the civil rights era, who initiated legal suits on behalf of hospitalized mental patients. The legal efforts had divergent results. A significant amount of litigation resulted in increasing the rights of hospitalized mental patients.

Respect for psychiatric expertise in legal, legislative and public opinion arenas was often diminished by critics calling into question the reliability and validity of diagnoses of mental disorders.

New Directions in Psychopathology

In the late 1950s there was a growing awareness among clinicians and researchers that the absence of objective, empirically based methods for describing psychopathology was limiting research efforts. Much of this concern appeared after the introduction of new psychopharmacologic agents and the need to assess their efficacy by controlled clinical trials. Many rating scales were developed in response to this need, including those by Lorr (1962), Hamilton (1960) and Overall (1962). Self-report instruments, such as the *Hopkins Symptom Checklist* (HSCL) (Derogatis et al., 1973) and the *Profile of Mood States* (POMS) (McNair, 1971) were also formulated. In addition, specific scales for depression and for anxiety were developed by Hamilton (1960), Beck (1969) and Zung (1965), among others.

These new advances in clinical psychopathology drew upon existing psychometric methodologies, particularly those developed for educational testing, and the new statistical techniques, including factor analysis and other multivariate methods. The availability of high-speed electronic computers in the early 1960s made possible the application of many statistical procedures previously too laborious to be undertaken manually.

In the 1950s and 1960s, these methods were applied to the description of symptoms of patients entering clinical drug trials and to assessment of the multidimensional nature of change produced by therapeutic intervention, particularly new drugs and community programs.

During the 1970s, psychometric methods were applied to problems of reliability and validity of categorical diagnostic categories. In this effort there has been a convergence of the neo-Kraepelinian approach (Robins & Guze, 1970, 1972), which emphasizes the importance of multiple classes of psychiatric illness, with the research methods and techniques of psychometrics and biostatistics. The first products of this collaboration were the *Research Diagnostic Criteria* (RDC) and the *Schizophrenia and Depression Schedule* (SADS) developed by Spitzer, Endicott and Robins (1975) as part of the NIMH Collaborative Psychobiology of Depression Project (Katz & Klerman, 1979). The RDC provided a compendium of operational criteria for 22 diagnostic classes. Based on the general approach of Robins and Guze (1970, 1972) and the Washington University/St. Louis group of neo-Kraepelinians, it was paired with a structured interview, the SADS. Together, the SADS-RDC provided major tools for systematic assessment of psychopathology and for assignment of patients to diagnostic classes. They were rapidly accepted as the standard clinical research procedures in the late 1970s in the United States.

Spitzer was appointed Chair of the APA Task Force to develop the DSM-III, and he and his associates developed operational criteria for many diagnostic classes (over 100 categories in all). They also devised a multiaxial system to aid diagnostic and treatment decisions. To test the reliability and clinical utility of the new DSM-III, a field trial involving over 400 psychiatrists was undertaken. Efforts to establish validity of diagnostic categories were also begun, based on principles articulated by Guze (1970) and Robins (1977), which emphasized external validation by correlation with laboratory studies, follow-up of clinical course and outcome, family and genetic associations, response to treatment, and social and economic factors.

The Neo-Kraepelinians

During the 1970s, a small group of neo-Kraepelinians emerged in American psychiatry and had major impact on research activity in psychiatric academic circles (Klerman, 1977) The neo-Kraepelinian point of view includes a number of normative propositions:

1) Psychiatry is a branch of medicine.

2) Psychiatric practice should be based on the results of scientific knowledge derived from rigorous empirical study (as contrasted with discursive and impressionistic interpretation).

3) A boundary exists between the normal and the sick and this boundary can be delineated reliably.

4) Within the domain of sickness, discrete mental illnesses exist and are not myths. Rather than a unitary phenomenon, mental illness consists of many disorders, and it is the task of scientific psychiatry, as well as other medical specialties, to investigate their etiology, diagnosis and treatment.

5) Psychiatry should treat individuals requiring medical care for mental illnesses, as opposed to those in need of assistance for problems-in-living and unhappiness.

6) Research and teaching should emphasize diagnosis and classification explicitly and intentionally.

7) Diagnostic criteria should be classified and research should validate the criteria for this classification.

8) Departments of psychiatry in medical schools should teach these criteria and not deprecate them, as has been the case for many years.

9) Research efforts directed at improving the reliability and validity of diagnosis and classification should use advanced quantitative research techniques.

10) Research in psychiatry should use modern scientific methodologies, especially from biology.

As is clear from these highly prescriptive propositions, the Neo-Kraepelinians were not interested in describing current psychiatric practice; they wanted to change it. Although the Neo-Kraepelinians tend to research genetic hypotheses for mental illness, a categorical approach is not, in my opinion, necessarily unique to biological psychiatry. For example, Freud and many of his early followers, such as Abraham (1927) and Glover, proposed a classification of mental illness based on psycho-sexual stages of development. In current research practice, however, most Neo-Kraepelinians emphasize the biological bases of mental disorders, and, as a group, they are neutral, ambivalent or at times even hostile to psychodynamic, interpersonal and social psychiatric approaches.

Theoretically, the concept of separate syndromes is compatible with behavioral and social psychiatric approaches. The writings, research efforts and clinical practice of the small but influential group of Neo-Kraepelinians in the States nevertheless remains closely identified with the biological school—part of a general trend in American psychiatry toward greater integration with general medicine. Although the impetus for this trend has come from several sources—professional, scientific, ideological and economic—one consequence has been a greater concern for the medical identity of U.S. psychiatry.

The initial statement of the Neo-Kraepelinian point of view appeared in the introduction to the textbook, *Clinical Psychiatry*, by Mayer-Gross, Slater and Roth, published in Britain in 1954. Strongly critical of psychoanalysis, psychotherapy, and social psychiatry, this book was a resounding and aggressive reaffirmation of the traditional Kraepelinian approach. In the United States, Neo-Kraepelinian activity originated at Washington University/St. Louis. Its early spokespersons were E. Robins, George Winokur and Sam Guze. Winokur has been active in familial-genetic studies of affective disorder, and Guze is best known for his research with Briquet's Syndrome and the reformulation of the category of "hysteria."

One impetus for these diagnostic efforts derives from psychopharmacology research and practice. The patterns of response to the major classes of therapeutic drugs has been striking in the degree to which

Kraepelin's diagnostic distinctions have been followed. Among the "functional" psychoses, schizophrenia, paranoia and other disorders of thinking respond to neuroleptics, while among the affective disorders, manic states respond to lithium and the depressions to tricyclics. The general pattern of response seems to follow the general outline of the major disorders. As the numbers of psychopharmacologic agents available grew in the 1960s and 1970s, efforts were undertaken to provide reliable and valid predictors of which types of patients were likely to respond to the various classes of drugs.

These new diagnostic procedures have also been effective in responding to the challenges from the antipsychiatrists and the labeling theorists. One of the main arguments put forth by the critics of psychiatry was the apparent low reliability of psychiatric diagnoses and the lack of validity for the categories. In response to this criticism, successful efforts were undertaken to better understand the sources of unreliability, and they have been located and analyzed: Efforts have been made and are continuing to be made to overcome reliability obstacles. For example, Fleiss, Spitzer and associates (1972) applied the statistic "kappa" to measure more accurately the degree of concordance among diagnosticians. In addition, training techniques have been developed using videotapes and case vignettes to aid in applying DSM-III operational criteria more precisely.

IV. The Contemporary Schools of American Psychiatry

The previous sections of this paper have described the major scientific and social forces within the profession and from the larger society, leading to the emergence of multiple schools of American psychiatry. Each of the major schools are now discussed with regard to their general background and scientific orientation, and their specific positions vis-à-vis diagnosis and classification of disorders.

The Decline and Rebirth of Biological Psychiatry

Biological psychiatry can trace its origins to mid-19th-century developments in European countries, notably France and Germany. The term "psychiatry" first appeared in the mid-19th century during the time of rapid emergence of other medical specialties. In the German-speaking countries, new advances in biology were applied to mental disorders. Bacteriology, pathology, physiology and biochemistry became separate scientific fields whose methods were quickly applied to psychiatric illnesses, often with striking success.

The tenets of the biological school were codified in the successive editions of Kraepelin's influential textbook (1919), which incorporated general principles for classifying mental disorders on the basis of etiology. Kraepelin also delineated dementia praecox and manic-depressive psychoses.

After the discoveries in 1911 that the Treponema organism was responsible for CNS syphilis, and in 1921 that pellagra was due to a deficiency in vitamin B6, the field of biological psychiatry went fallow: New discoveries were uncommon and scientific work became undistinguished. At the same time, the available somatic treatments seemed inhumane, with many biological psychiatrists showing an overenthusiasm for interventions such as colostomy, adrenalectomy and excision of teeth, justified by notions of autoinfection and other unsubstantiated theories. Psychosurgery was performed widely without adequate evidence as to its efficacy or safety. By the end of World War II, biological psychiatry had become identified with therapeutic insensitivity and scientific mediocrity.

A resurgence of biological psychiatry occurred in the mid-1950s with the development of new psychopharmacologic agents, particularly the phenothiazines, the effects of which were to create a therapeutic revolution and to change the nature of psychiatric institutionalization. With the development of lithium, the tricyclics and MAO inhibitors for affective disorders, wide, controlled testing of these agents in clinical practice was begun.

Efforts of laboratory investigators to understand the mode of actions of the new drugs witnessed a renewed interest in relating psychiatry to neurobiology. The U.S. leader of these investigations was Seymour Kety and his associates at the NIMH Intramural Program at Bethesda, Maryland.

Techniques from enzymology, neuropharmacology, neurophysiology and neurochemistry were rapidly employed to understand the CNS action of the new psychotropic agents and to elucidate possible biological abnormalities in schizophrenic, manic-depressive and other patient groups.

Developments in psychiatric genetics, following upon the discoveries of molecular biology, opened up an additional area of investigation of the etiology of psychiatric illness. Kety and his associates were the leaders in these explorations as well. Their elegant Danish cross-fostering studies (1968) permitted the first demonstration of the interaction of genetic and environmental factors in the etiology of schizophrenia.

As has been noted, clinical responses to the new drugs revealed patterns that followed classic categorization of major disorders. The therapeutic efficacy of these psychopharmacologic agents stimulated a search for clinical predictors of response for diagnostic subclasses. For example, the clinical picture of endogenous depression has been found to predict response to tricyclics, and attempts are now underway to develop diagnostic criteria for "atypical depressions" that respond to MAO inhibitors.

Although clinical psychopathological features have had considerable utility in predicting response to drugs, the almost total reliance on behavioral and symptomatic observations for clinical decisions has prompted dissatisfaction. In the context of this dissatisfaction, current efforts to develop biological laboratory tests are increasing.

At the present time, the biological school in psychiatry is closest to the mainstream of general medicine. Its proponents are a minority within the practitioners in the United States, based on surveys of the self-defined identity of psychiatrists, with a higher proportion in academic and research settings (Armor & Klerman, 1968). Although its adherents are relatively few in number among clinicians, the quality of research in biological psychiatry and the promise of future knowledge have been dramatic. Increasing evidence for the efficacy of psychopharmacologic agents, based on results of controlled clinical trials, has produced a greater willingness of practitioners to use drugs in the treatment of patients who previously would have had recourse only to much less rigorously tested somatic treatments or to some form of psychotherapy. These accomplishments have captured the imagination not only of psychiatrists, but also of other physicians, mental health professionals, the public-at-large and government policy makers.

The Emergence of the Psychoanalytic School

Hale (1971) and other historians have documented the rapid infusion of psychoanalysis into American psychiatry and intellectual thought after Freud lectured at Clark University in Worcester, Massachusetts, in 1908. The psychiatric scene in the United States at the turn of the century was characterized by crises in the three prominent modes of treatment of mental illness: the custodial nature of the institutional area was woefully inadequate and support for the "asylum" was in decline; the somatic mode was employed by neurologists increasingly frustrated in their attempts to deal with problems involving the emotions; and the new psychotherapies used eclectic investigation of suggestion and reeducation techniques.

This state of dissatisfaction provided fertile ground for the acceptance of Freud's concepts and methods involving the unconscious. The leading psychologists and psychotherapists of the time, most particularly William James and Morton Prince, accepted Freud's theories of infantile sexuality and repression as they sought to understand more fully the nature of psychological conflict. The intellectual network that included James, Prince, Boris Sidis, the neurologist James Jackson Putnam, Adolf Meyer and others helped provide acceptance of the psychoanalytic movement in the medical academic centers of Boston, Baltimore and New York.

Freud's ideas attracted physicians outside as well as inside the psychoanalytic movement, such as William Alanson White, director of St. Elizabeth's Hospital in Washington, DC, who had learned from Meyer to study patients' "mental makeup" and life experience. Psychiatric hospitals and medical schools began to employ and teach psychoanalytic techniques, influential medical textbooks sympathetic to psychoanalysis appeared, and between the time of Freud's visit in 1909 and the end of World War I in 1918, the number of interested physicians had markedly increased across the country.

The pervasive influence of Adolf Meyer, the most influential psychiatrist on the American scene between the two World Wars, was also important. Because psychoanalysis emphasized psychological and environmental factors rather than heredity and somatic disturbances, Meyer initially found Freud's approach stimulating in his own explorations and critiques of dementia praecox, as well as in his psychobiological efforts to break through a rigid body/mind dualism. Although he never fully embraced psychoanalytic concepts or methods, in 1930 he stated that Freud had organized and articulated psychological tenets more telling than any in the previous 30 years, in terms close to the "heart of passion and conflict" (Hale, 1971).

The social climate in the United States also nurtured the belief in cure of mental illness through treatment focused on psychological conflict, repression, childhood experience and dreams. The psychoanalytic approach came to be regarded as having clinical value and theoretical significance. Garnering support from diverse professional, academic and lay sources, psychoanalysis established an influential position in American psychiatry and culture.

During the early history of the psychoanalytic movement, its theorists and clinicians accepted the basic Kraepelinian views of nosology. Moreover, in many ways, Freud was the "Kraepelin of the psychoneuroses," having written many of the original descriptions of anxiety neuroses, obsessive-compulsive states, conversion hysteria and phobia. Freud himself wrote a number of important papers on the distinction between neuroses and psychoses, basing the distinction on a number of criteria: (1) regression from secondary to primary thinking, (2) different levels in fixation of psychosexual development, (3) the influence of narcissism, and (4) loss of reality testing in psychoses and retention of reality in neuroses.

Many early psychoanalytic workers adopted a nosologic model that related the individual psychoses, neuroses and other mental disorders to fixations at specific states of psychosexual development. Abraham (1927) and Fenichel (1945) were explicit about this model and their writings included charts in which connections are drawn between particular states of child development and the predisposition to specific adult disorders.

This model, however, became increasingly untenable in the 1940s, when alternative models were attempted in order to incorporate and apply the new concepts of child development, particularly those proposed by Anna Freud.

Social Psychiatry

Adolf Meyer's psychobiology extended the Darwinian principle of biological adaptation to include the human organism's psychic adaptation to its social environment. In Meyer's view, psychiatric illness represented an attempt, or usually the failure of an attempt, by the individual to cope with environmental demands. In his writings, however, Meyer was vague as to the specific psychopathogenic characteristics of the social environment or how they were related to the emergence of specific mental illnesses. However, his students, especially Lemkau, Pasamanick, Rennie and Leighton launched the school of social psychiatry with their field studies of social epidemiology in the United States after World War II.

Four aspects of the social environment became the focus of social psychiatric interest: social class, stress, civilization and urbanization, and the social structure of mental institutions:

(1) *Social class.* The observation that certain mental illnesses were more prevalent in lower social classes was reported at a time of national concern with poverty and other consequences of inequality in the United States. This influential line of research began with the work of the Chicago school of sociology, particularly by Faris and Dunham (1939), who used ecological methods to demonstrate differences in hospitalization associated with social class. Subsequently, Hollingshead and Redlich (1958) studied the prevalence of treated mental illness in New Haven, Connecticut. Although their work has been criticized for its failure to distinguish adequately between incidence and prevalence and for its restriction of the sample to treated cases, they nevertheless demonstrated a strong relationship between lower

social class and schizophrenia. Moreover, they documented the powerful influence of social class on availability of treatment resources and health-seeking behavior.

(2) *Stress.* During World War II, an extensive social science research program was conducted by the U.S. Army that included efforts relating neurotic symptoms to combat stress (Stouffer, 1950). Although military personnel had passed extensive Selective Service medical and psychiatric screenings prior to induction, some among them nonetheless developed psychiatric symptoms during combat. Researchers thus concluded that combat neuroses were precipitated by stress rather than caused by predisposing vulnerability.

The thesis that mental illness in the military was due to precipitating stress factors led to many studies on the relationship between psychosocial life events and mental disorders in civilian life. Holmes and Rahe (1967), for example, initiated a series of studies on the role of various stressors in increasing the relative risk of becoming ill; natural disasters (such as hurricanes and floods), life events (such as grief or loss of a job), and economic changes (such as the closing of an industrial plant) were selected as known to increase risk of medical and mental illness.

(3) *Civilization and urbanization.* The earliest speculations as to the causes of mental illness arose during the Enlightenment when mental illness was viewed as the result of civilization. Rousseau's concept of the "happy savage" was reflected in the epidemiologic hypothesis that mental illness does not occur in the natural (i.e., uncivilized) state of man, an hypothesis that Srole and Fischer (1980) refer to as the "paradise lost" doctrine of mental illness. This romantic view of primitive societies rested on the assumption that these societies do not have psychoses, an assumption contradicted by cross-cultural research demonstrating that mental illnesses, including psychosis, occur widely throughout both literate and nonliterate societies (Murphy, 1976).

Goldhammer and Marshall (1953) also tested this hypothesis using data on rates of mental hospitalizations in Massachusetts. Their research indicated that when the rates are corrected for the changing age distribution of the population, no trend toward increased hospitalization because of psychoses during any particular time period could be documented for patients below the age of 50 since the 19th century.

Closely related to civilization as a focal point for social psychiatric investigation is urbanization associated with view that urban social life has adverse mental health effects. This epidemiological thesis predicts that mental illness will be more prevalent in urban than rural communities.

Srole and Fischer (1980) recently tested this hypothesis in a follow-up study of persons interviewed in the Midtown Manhattan study of 1954. When controlled for age and decades of Manhattan living, more recent birth cohorts showed *better* mental health compared to the earlier generation. This finding was due mainly to an improvement in the mental health of the "new breed of women" emerging in recent years.

Parallel to the 1954 Midtown Manhattan study has been the important study of Leighton and associates in Nova Scotia (1963). Their work tested the thesis that rapid social change, particularly from a rural economy to an industrial social economic structure, results in breakdown of social cohesion and increases social disorganization, reflected in increasing rates of mental illness. Their concept of social disintegration bears many similarities to Durkheim's *anomie* (1951).

(4) *The social structure of mental institutions.* After World War II, a number of successful collaborations were undertaken between psychiatrists and sociologists to investigate the social, psychological and institutional characteristics of mental hospitals. These studies demonstrated the adverse impact of the mental hospital social structure on clinical outcome. Excessive bureaucracy, hierarchical authority structure, the power exerted by nonprofessionals and the pervasive role of ideology were emphasized. These findings revived interest in the moral therapy of the early 19th century, with its emphasis on the individual and the role of the institutional environment in actively promoting recovery.

The results of these investigations questioned whether much, or even all, of the clinical features associated with schizophrenia and other chronic psychoses were due to the intrinsic nature of the illness or to the depersonalizing and dependency-producing features of the social environment of the institution.

In England, the concept of "institutional neuroses" was proposed to account for these effects. In the United States, Gruenberg (1966) identified a "social breakdown syndrome" from the effect of the social environment on the course of illness, particularly those outcomes with deterioration. In part based on these studies, many attempts were made to reform mental hospitals. American psychiatrists adopted many of the techniques originating in the United Kingdom, including "open door" policies, day treatment programs, and efforts at social and vocational rehabilitation. Innovation along these lines has been less than prominent in the past decade, during which attention has shifted from the hospital to the community as the main locus of treatment.

The closing of mental hospitals, similar to the widespread closing of tuberculosis hospitals during the 1950s, has remained an unrealized hope. Rather, community placement and deinstitutionalization have often witnessed continuing chronicity and social disability among patients, indicating that a considerable proportion of chronic social disability is attributable to the illness rather than to the adverse effects of the institutional social structure.

The social psychiatry school made two main contributions to research: (1) Its efforts enlarged the scope of psychiatric research concerns by focusing on institutions and large populations; and (2) it brought social science theory and methodology into the field of psychiatric research. Although psychiatric epidemiologic efforts have broadened the class of relevant independent variables (the causal risk factors) associated with mental illness, students of social epidemiology have paid relatively less attention to the dependent variables (the specific mental disorders).

There was, in fact, a tendency in many epidemiologic studies after World War II to depreciate specific diagnoses and to rely upon unidimensional disability and mental impairment scales (Weissman and Klerman, 1978). This tendency was reversed with the application of the *Research Diagnostic Criteria* (RDC) and other new techniques in community surveys. NIMH developed the Epidemiologic Catchment Area (ECA) program which involved community surveys of large samples of patients at multiple sites using a structured interview, and the *Diagnostic Interview Schedule* (DIS) formulated by Robins (1981), which allows for diagnostic assessment consistent with DSM-III categories. These efforts have provided a rapprochement between the new emphasis on diagnostic categories and the theoretical and methodological advances in sampling and measurement of social risk factors developed by social psychiatric researchers.

The Behavioral School

A behavioral school of psychiatry emerged in North America in the 1960s. Although its intellectual and scientific origins are to be found in the work of Pavlov and Schenechov in Russia and the early writings of Watson on behaviorism in the United States, the main theoretical support for contemporary behaviorism is derived from the work of B.F. Skinner.

The growth of behaviorism as a psychiatric school was associated with considerable controversy and tension between M.D. psychiatrists and Ph.D. clinical psychologists. Most behavior therapists and researchers hold Ph.D.s, although a sizable and influential minority are behaviorally oriented psychiatrists.

Whereas the main focus of behavior therapy, research and practice has been on the treatment of symptomatic states, such as phobias, obsessive-compulsive states or sexual dysfunction, a number of theoretical and ideological aspects of behavior therapy bear upon issues in nosology, diagnosis and classification. On the whole, behaviorists are skeptical of diagnostic categories and phenomena that cannot be directly observed, such as intrapsychic conflicts or unconscious mental processes. They have, thus, been highly critical of psychodynamic concepts and similarly skeptical about the standard view of personality states or personality disorders as enduring.

The behaviorists' emphasis on directly observable behavior, rather than inner mental states, has contributed to their extensive use of rating scales, self-report methods and patients' diaries. Psychometric techniques that have been developed, usually rating scales, have been used to quantify the magnitude of symptoms, such as phobias and obsessive-compulsive behavior. Much less attention, however, has been given to problems of differential diagnosis or to a syndromal approach.

London (1971) called attention to the strong ideological components in the behavioral approach. He argued that the claims by behaviorists that learning theory provides a scientific basis for clinical practice, as well as their attack on mental entities, appear to him to be related more to the need of behavior therapists to separate themselves from their psychoanalytic and psychiatric colleagues than to a large body of directly relevant scientific evidence.

V. Research Approaches to the Diagnosis and Classification of Selected Disorders

Having described the historical background leading to the development of multiple schools within U.S. psychiatry, I now describe briefly how these schools apply their principles and methods to issues in the diagnosis and classification of selected disorders. In the context of general trends in American psychiatry, I focus on recent efforts, based on the Third Edition of the *Diagnostic and Statistical Manual* (DSM-III).

Schizophrenia and Related Conditions

During and following World War II, American psychiatry adopted an expanded definition of schizophrenia. In part this was due to the strong influence in teaching institutions of Bleuler's concept of schizophrenia, which was broader than Kraepelin's dementia praecox.

As the concept of schizophrenia broadened, it came to encompass all nonorganic psychoses. American patients diagnosed as schizophrenic overlapped with patients diagnosed by European psychiatry as having manic, schizoaffective and depressive psychoses. Moreover, the expanded diagnostic category of schizophrenia came to include many nonpsychotic states, characterized by chronic difficulties in social adjustment, impairment of personality functions and regressive phenomena, even though these states might not involve impairment of reality testing or loss of higher mental functions.

In the 1960s, a number of efforts led to a reevaluation of the broad concept of schizophrenia and the movement toward a narrower definition. These include:

1) *The U.S.-U.K. Diagnostic Project.* In the late 1950s, M. Kramer, head of the NIMH Biometrics Program, took note of the marked discrepancy between the United States and the United Kingdom regarding the numbers (in rates per 100,000) of patients hospitalized and diagnosed as schizophrenic or depressive in each country. He questioned the extent to which these statistics reflected true differences in the incidence and prevalence of the disorders or were due to diagnostic differences. Kramer (1969) and Zubin (1969) at the New York State Psychiatric Institute enlisted colleagues at Maudsley Hospital, notably Wing and Cooper (1974), to launch the U.S.-U.K. joint project. Collaborative research teams were organized in London and in New York, and standardized interview instruments were developed, indexing Wing's *Present State Examination* (PSE). This study documented that the U.S.-U.K. differences in hospitalization rates were mainly due to the different criteria employed in making diagnoses: The British psychiatrists were found to be more likely to diagnose affective disorders for cases that U.S. psychiatrists diagnosed as schizophrenic.

2) *The advent of lithium.* Support for a narrower diagnostic concept of schizophrenia was provided by the efficacy of lithium for bipolar patients. This clinical advance permitted a reduction in the number of patients diagnosed as schizophrenic by removing those with manic symptoms, particularly excitement and overactivity, from the large psychiatric group. In addition, the reports that some patients clinically diagnosed as schizophrenic or paranoid also responded to lithium prompted further reassessment of diagnostic practices.

3) *The development of standardized criteria.* The diagnostic criteria first described by Feighner and the St. Louis group (1972) were found applicable to several research efforts requiring more specific means for distinguishing patient classes. These criteria were later incorporated and expanded into the *Research Diagnostic Criteria* (RDC) developed by Spitzer, Endicott and Robins (1975) for the NIMH Psychobiology Program (Katz & Klerman, 1979) and then into the DSM-III and the DSM-III-R.

4) *The WHO International Pilot Study for Schizophrenia.* The IPSS demonstrated the feasibility of employing standardized criteria in many countries, as well as documenting the similarities and differences between U.S. diagnostic practices and those of other countries (WHO, 1978).

With DSM-III, the U.S. nomenclature shifted to a narrower definition of schizophrenia. In fact, there is now concern that the DSM-III, especially the requirements of a 6-month duration, may be too narrow. As has been noted, the psychoanalytic and interpersonal schools came to deemphasize the descriptive Kraepelinian formulations of psychopathology. Rather than focusing on psychotic manifestations of delusions and hallucinations as necessary criteria for diagnosis of schizophrenia, the patient's inner conflicts and defences, family patterns, interpersonal relations, and social functioning were emphasized.

Researchers and practitioners of the interpersonal school continue to emphasize psychosocial and psychotherapeutic factors with the schizophrenic patient and/or the family, although these efforts are less prominent than in the 1950s and 1960s. Through the formulation of multidimensional assessments that include social adjustment, family relations, personality and occupational factors, and community integration, their work has broadened the range of outcomes to include more than changes in symptoms.

After the studies on New Haven reported by Hollingshead and Redlich (1958), social psychiatric researchers focused their efforts in the 1960s on the role of social class in relation to schizophrenia. This line of research seems to have reached an impasse, with relatively little resolution of the controversy as to whether the social class differences among individuals with the illness reflect true differences in incidence and prevalence, or differences in access to and utilization of treatment facilities. Another related, persistent issue also remains unsolved: Does the accumulation of treated cases in the lower socioeconomic classes reflect social drift within and/or across generations due to adverse consequences of illness? Or does it represent the consequences of pathogenic features of lower socioeconomic class experience?

The behavioral school has paid relatively little attention to diagnostic issues in schizophrenia. Behaviorists have experimented with reinforcement schedules and token economics used in the inpatient treatment setting and with social skills training useful for rehabilitation, particularly in patients' transition to community living after discharge. Lieberman at UCLA and Camillio State Hospital and Paul in Illinois are prominent in these efforts.

The American fascination with the broad definition of schizophrenia was associated with little interest in other "functional psychoses." Occasional reports have appeared on paranoid psychoses, and the debate continues as to whether paranoid states are to be subsumed under schizophrenia or should be regarded as a distinct diagnostic group. The schizoaffective diagnosis has not gained wide acceptance in U.S. clinical practice and the studies devoted to its description or validation remain relatively few. The "third psychosis," schizoaffective states and cycloid psychoses, have slowly gained attention among researchers (Winokur, McCabe, Tsuang and Clayton, Guze).

The Affective Disorders

DSM-II and the ICD-8 did not group the affective disorders as one diagnostic class, but separated them into the psychotic and neurotic categories. The recent trend in the United States has been to group the affective disorders together as a diagnostic class, a tendency that has minimized, but not eliminated, the distinction between psychotic and neurotic forms. This trend is clear in research employing the RDC, as well as in the formulation of the large category comprising all affective disorders in the DSM-III and DSM-III-R. The creation of this category with several subclasses was based on the large body of research during the 1960s and 1970s on psychopathologic, biological and therapeutic aspects of depression and mania.

The concept of bipolar affective disorder has been widely accepted for its clinical utility in predicting positive response to lithium and adverse response to tricyclics, and has proven a strong spur to research on genetic and biochemical aspects of the disorders.

The concept of unipolar depression is less well accepted. All that is not bipolar is not unipolar. DSM-III does not specify a unipolar category.

The concept of neurotic depression has been radically revised. Defined in terms of multiplicity of factors, including long-term personality difficulties, precipitation by acute stress, underlying unconscious conflicts, as well as others, the DSM-II diagnosis of psychoneurotic depressive reaction was among the most common diagnoses in clinical practice. Research and clinical experience have increasingly questioned the utility and validity of this concept (Klerman et al., 1979; Akiskal, 1978), contributing to the deletion of the diagnostic category in the DSM-III.

Considerable research on the role of life events as possible precipitants of various forms of affective disorder has led to a questioning of the validity of a separate category of "reactive" or "situational" depression (Hirschfeld, 1980). Although life events may increase the risk for a wide variety of disorders, including schizophrenic and medical conditions as well as affective disorders, life events as unique precipitants of any clinical form of affective disorder is increasingly in question.

Attention to endogenous depression has increased. R. Kuhn observed that patients with endogenous depressions responded to tricyclics (Kuhn, 1958). Factor-analytic studies were initially undertaken by Kiloh and Garside (1963) and others in the Newcastle group. Numerous replications of the factor-analytic studies in the United States (Mendels & Cochrane, 1968) identified a cluster of symptoms including early morning wakening, loss of interest in activities and pleasure, loss of appetite, loss of weight and psychomotor change, whether in the direction of agitation or retardation. Evidence has accrued that this symptom cluster is both independent of precipitating life events and highly predictive of response to ECT and to tricyclic antidepressants.

A major advance in classification of affective disorders was the proposal by Robins and Guze (1972) to separate primary and secondary depressions when using the criterion of temporal coexistence of other psychiatric conditions, particularly schizophrenia and alcoholism. Klerman and Barrett (1973) proposed that the diagnosis of secondary depression be extended to include conditions associated with preexisting medical disorder or drug reactions. The occurrence of mania secondary to medical conditions has led to a proposal for the diagnostic category of secondary mania (Krauthammer & Klerman, 1978).

The large number of ambulatory patients with symptoms of both anxiety and depression generates nosological confusion and diagnostic uncertainty. In clinical practice, the coexistence of both symptoms tends to be diagnosed as anxiety disorder, most often treated with antianxiety drugs of the chlordiazepoxide series. However, a number of studies have questioned the therapeutic efficacy of this class of drugs in depressions. It is possible that a separate category for anxiety-depression will appear in future nomenclatures.

Although use of the classic psychotic-neurotic distinction has diminished, the presence of delusions and other manifestations of psychoses is of clinical and therapeutic importance. Patients with delusions and hallucinations respond poorly to tricyclic antidepressants. The nosologic significance of this finding for the classification of affective disorders is still uncertain. The importance for treatment decisions in these cases, however, has gained increasing attention. Uncertainty still exists as to whether patients with delusions as a feature of their depressions are best treated with a combination of tricyclics or with ECT.

Disorders Previously Considered "Neurotic" Conditions

The decision to eliminate "neurotic conditions" as a separate category in DSM-III has generated considerable controversy. Many members of the clinical and academic community, particularly those influenced by psychodynamic thinking, have reacted negatively to this decision. The rationale governing this change was based on dissatisfaction with the vagueness of criteria for separating psychotic from neurotic conditions. Also, more significantly, there was concern that the terms "neurotic" and "psychotic" had become confounded with etiological presumptions—psychotic conditions were presumed of constitutional, genetic or biochemical origin, while neurotic conditions resulted from environmental, personality or psychosocial factors.

Within the group of conditions categorized diagnostically as "neurotic" in DSM-II, and still grouped as such in the ICD-9, the individual disorders remain relatively unchanged, although their grouping has been changed. Obsessive-compulsive and generalized anxiety disorders are subsumed in DSM-III under the larger category of anxiety disorders. Within this category, panic disorder and agoraphobia have been separated from other phobias. The justification for this change rests not only on differences in subjective experience and clinical course, but also on differences in treatment response. In clinical trials, agoraphobia and panic attacks have been shown to be relatively unresponsive to antianxiety drugs of the benzodiazepoxide type other than alprazolam, but responsive to tricyclic antidepressants and MAO inhibitors.

Behavior treatment has proved increasingly effective with agoraphobic patients in the United States and in the United Kingdom. However, many English thinkers do not accept Klein's distinction between panic disorder and generalized anxiety, and the division of agoraphobia from other forms of phobias. Further research will be required to reconcile these differences (Roth & Argyle, 1988).

Another controversial new diagnostic category is somatization disorder. This term derives from research by Guze and his associates (1972) on Briquet's Syndrome, and was proposed in an attempt to reduce the confusion and emotionally charged responses to diagnosis of "hysteria."

DSM-III retains the category of disassociative disorders and allows for separate diagnosis of the various forms (amnesia, fugue, multiple personality and depersonalization). Although these conditions are seen infrequently, the psychopathology is often dramatic, and increased understanding is important for theory and research efforts.

The behavioral school has been most attentive to the phobias, obsessive-compulsive states and forms of psychosocial dysfunction, with which behavioral psychotherapy has been most successful. Although the development of behavioral interventions depends in large part on delineation of psychopathologic states based on symptoms, there is a strong antinosologic bias within the behavioral school, and research patients have been selected on the basis of predominant behavior and manifest symptoms, such as phobias or sexual dysfunction. However, as the range of application of behavioral psychotherapy has expanded, some rapprochement with nosological diagnosis has begun to occur, and investigators using behavioral techniques are increasingly using structured interviews and diagnostic algorithms in selecting research patients (Barlow et al., 1986).

Personality Disorders

Recent American trends with regard to the diagnostic classification of personality disorders have been reviewed comprehensively by Frances (1980) and also by Vaillant and Perry (1980). Both papers discuss a number of important trends on the American scene with regard to nosology and research of these disorders.

Dimensions of the disordered personality and the healthy individual are both similar and vastly different. While in some instances the clinical disorders (obsessive-compulsive states) appear to be quantitative extensions of healthy mechanisms, in other instances they appear to be discontinuous from normal behavior, as in the case of the antisocial personality. In the case of psychodynamic ego, their manifestations are modified adaptively in healthy individuals and are greatly different from manifestations seen as clinical conditions meriting treatment. Yet they are the same defenses.

Most researchers on personality in psychology use dimensional assessment methods relying heavily on data from self-report and interviews to produce quantitative measures of traits, attributes, and characteristics. With the advent of computers, multivariate statistical techniques, particularly discriminate function and factor analysis, have been applied to many of the older personality inventories, in particular those developed by Cattell (1957), Murray (1953) and the MMPI. The attempt in these efforts has been to develop psychometrically pure measures, not only of individual personality traits, but also of the clustering together of various traits into patterns, types or constellations. As yet, the relation of these approaches to the clinical disorders remains relatively unclear theoretically, empirically and clinically.

DSM-III included a number of new personality disorders derived mainly from the clinical experience of the psychoanalytic and interpersonal schools. The two conditions in DSM-III reflecting this influence most are "narcissistic personality disorder" and "borderline personality disorder." Narcissistic personality disorder is based on concepts of American psychoanalytic writing and practice articulated by Kohut and his associates (1966, 1971). The reliability, validity and correlates of narcissistic personality disorder are being systematically studied.

The borderline personality disorder was originally described by Knight (1953), who delineated borderline schizophrenic states in a similar manner to prior descriptions of "latent" or "ambulatory" schizophrenia. Knight's ideas also contributed to the extensions of the definition of schizophrenia. In the mid-1960s, a gradual shift in focus occurred with the publication of a number of papers focused on enduring personality features rather than the transient psychotic states. The earlier concept of borderline schizophrenia with transient psychiatric states has been incorporated in DSM-III as "schizotypic personality disorder," a disorder presumably different from the borderline personality disorder. Efforts have been made to apply quantitative psychometric approaches for the diagnosis and treatment of the borderline personality disorder, particularly in the work of Gunderson and Singer (1975), Grinker (1977), and Perry and Klerman (1978).

A number of the classic personality disorders remained relatively unchanged in DSM-III: paranoid personality disorder, schizoid personality disorder, histrionic personality disorder (previously called hysterical personality), antisocial personality disorder (previously called sociopathy), compulsive personality disorder and dependent personality disorder. Evidence for the diagnostic validity of dependent personality and passive personality disorders remains relatively meager.

The decision to retain histrionic personality disorder (hysterical personality disorder) is the subject of continuing controversy and has come under increasing fire from the feminist movement, which criticizes the criteria as reflecting a male definition of femininity. The stereotypic characterization of hysteria remains a source of contention, despite attempts to validate the disorder by clinical and psychological studies.

In the opinion of most clinicians and investigators, the multiaxial approach of DSM-III for the diagnosis of personality disorders represents a major advance, corresponding more to the diversity of patient characteristics occurring in clinical experience than is usually included in official diagnostic nomenclature. Nonetheless, further work on Axis II is required in order to include disturbances of personality functioning not meeting the criteria for a "disorder," but of clinical importance.

Disorders in Children

One of the first subspecialties in American psychiatry, child psychiatry arose from efforts to diagnose and evaluate children, especially delinquents involved with the juvenile justice system, to determine their physical and mental needs as well as legal disposition. The field thus began in the court and the clinic by way of the child guidance movement, pioneered by William Healey, founder and director of the Juvenile Psychopathic Institute in Chicago, the first child guidance center in the country. The public interest in child development that grew during the Progressive era and the fiscal support of the Commonwealth Fund fostered a network of child guidance demonstration clinics that developed a team approach providing psychiatric care for children and social casework for parents.

The influence of Adolf Meyer, with its emphasis on the interrelation of experience, habit and adaptation, along with the psychosexual development theories of psychoanalysis introduced in the United States in the first decades of the 20th century, provided the theoretical basis for new guidance center programs.

The current subspecialty of child psychiatry reflects, in many important ways, its early beginnings in the child guidance centers where emphasis was on the child's early experience, parental childrearing practices, the socioenvironmental influences on formation of symptoms, and psychotherapy of the child and parents as the major therapeutic intervention.

The special section in DSM-III devoted to disorders of children and adolescents includes several innovations, the most prominent being operational criteria, expansion of the multiaxial system first developed in child psychiatry by the WHO working group, and expansion of the classification by the Group for the Advancement of Psychiatry (GAP).

Agreement regarding the category of mental retardation exists among all schools of psychiatry. The DSM-III incorporates the terminology and nosology of the American Association on Mental Deficiency. Specific changes and innovative features may, however, require further refinement before acceptance of other more problematic categories occurs. In DSM-III, "minimum brain dysfunction" (MBD) and "hyperkinetic learning disability" were renamed Attentional Deficit Disorder (ADD). The validity of this disorder has been the source of much controversy, not only on scientific grounds, but also because of the possible abuse of this diagnosis among children from minority and poverty backgrounds. Moreover, there is a question as to whether these manifestations can be established as symptomatic of some defect in attention, as implied in the new term for the disorder.

A large group of conditions are grouped together as "conduct disorder." This category remains vaguely described and a subject of uncertainty, inasmuch as the major manifestations usually involve social maladjustment, most often presented in the school setting. Considerably greater specificity occurs in the area of eating disorders and the development of operational criteria for anorexia nervosa and bulimia.

A new category, "separation anxiety," groups together manifestations previously referred to as "school refusal" and "school phobia." Here, as with the attention deficit disorder, there is a presumption of an underlying psychic mechanism—in this case a special form of anxiety—for these behaviors. Diagnosis is thus made on this basis, as well as on specific behavioral manifestations. To this extent, the DSM-III deviates from its own precepts, indicating that further work in these areas is required.

Another addition—"identity disorder" in adolescence—is derived from the writings of Erikson (1968) and incorporates a widely discussed developmental concept derived from the psychoanalytic school.

The reaction of child psychiatry clinicians to DSM-III in the United States has been very mixed. In the early stages of the development of the DSM-III, the clinicians objected that the criteria emphasized descriptive psychopathology unduly and paid insufficient attention to personality dynamics and developmental processes. Despite the controversy and criticisms, however, the development of the DSM-III has provided considerable stimulus to research on diagnostic evaluations and efforts to establish the validity of many of the newer disorders, as well as to clarify the criteria for the more traditional disorders.

Advances in biological psychiatry have been slowly extended to infancy, childhood and adolescence. Most evident are those in the areas of mental retardation and the emotional states, particularly depression, and the various movement disorders. With regard to the latter group, Tourette's disorder, in particular, has been the subject of considerable research on family background and response to medication. The influence of biological research techniques is also seen in the distinction between sleepwalking disorder and sleep terror disorder, and the incorporation of research findings using sleep EEG.

The influence of developmental psychology and behavioral techniques are seen in the classification of criteria for reading disorders and related problems in language, arithmetic and other areas of learning disability. These are now incorporated in Axis II of DSM-III, which focuses on developmental disorders of childhood and adolescence.

Psychiatric Disorders of Old Age

Geriatric psychiatry has recently emerged as a subspecialty in the U.S. The quality of research and clinical practice has improved considerably, in part because of the attention focused on the increasing proportion of the population reaching old age and their impact on the health care and social services systems.

Whereas DSM-III has a special category of disorders that manifest in infancy, childhood and adolescence, no such category exists for the elderly. The major syndromes associated with aging include dementia and delirium, usually involving CNS or medical illnesses.

Syndromes of dementia and delirium and the various disorders associated with them are grouped in the DSM-III category of organic mental disorders. Among the advances in this area is the delineation of a separate category for multiinfarct dementia, representing a modification of previous thinking. In the past, many of the dementias associated with aging were attributed to generalized arteriosclerosis. It is now agreed that the cardiovascular events of thrombosis and hemorrhage resulting in infarction, rather than the diffuse vascular disease per se, contribute significantly to organic mental disorder.

Alzheimer's disease and Pick's disease, conditions previously regarded separately, are now grouped as primary degenerative dementia. This condition is often called primary dementia of the Alzheimer type.

Considerable advances in neuropathology and molecular biology have been made with regard to primary degenerative dementia. Neurofibrillary tangles have been identified as a specific neuropathologic finding, and their chemical composition is under investigation. Clinically, a tendency toward diffuse ventricular enlargement with cerebral atrophy has been documented using CAT scan techniques. Recently Position Emission Tomography (PET) has indicated a pervasive decrease in overall brain activity in patients with Alzheimer's disease as well as a general correlation between the severity of cognitive impairment with reduction in brain functioning. Whether or not CAT scan and PET scan techniques will become sufficiently established to become routine diagnostic procedures remains uncertain.

Disorders Related to Alcohol

Although research on the psychiatric consequences of alcohol ingestion was undertaken in the late 19th century, since the 1930s, with the end of Prohibition, there has been longstanding tension between psychiatry and the newly emergent field of alcoholism. American psychiatry in the first half of the 20th century paid relatively little attention to alcoholism. Psychoanalytically oriented approaches had interpreted alcohol abuse and resultant medical and psychiatric problems as behavioral consequences of pervasive antecedent personality disorders, drawing attention to personality features such as latent homosexuality, dependency, passivity, orality and inability to tolerate anxiety, depression and frustration. These personality formulations have generated negative reactions among many alcoholic patients and those in the alcoholism organizations such as Alcoholics Anonymous (AA) and the National Council on Alcoholism (NCA).

The DSM-III diagnostic nomenclature incorporates the recommendation of numerous WHO committees that have proposed the term "alcohol dependency" in place of imprecise terms such as "addiction." The concept of "alcohol dependence" represents extension into the field of alcoholism concepts originally developed with regard to drug abuse. In DSM-III, alcohol dependence is differentiated from "alcohol abuse," the latter being characterized by excessive use of alcohol with associated social, psychological and health impairments. Epidemiologic studies have indicated a high prevalence of both alcohol dependence and alcohol abuse in the United States and have identified important risk factors in modes of use and abuse by sex, age and social background.

Recent research in biological psychiatry has emphasized the role of genetic and familial factors. In their Danish study, D. Goodwin and associates (1976) employed cross-rearing techniques to disentangle genetic from environmental influences on the adopted offspring of alcoholic patients identified through the Danish case registry. They interpret the findings as suggesting a strong genetic influence.

In a parallel fashion, Winokur and associates (1970) have drawn attention to the high co-morbidity of alcoholism and depression, and suggested possible common predisposition. The co-morbidity of alcoholism and depression has been noted in clinical settings, particularly since the application of standardized interview techniques such as the SADS, DIS and standardized diagnostic criteria such as the RDC and DSM-III. The high ratio of males to females among alcoholics is attributed in some interpersonal and social psychiatric circles to the social channeling of subclinical depressive/dysphoric features. The hypothesis is that men treat their dysphoric symptoms with alcohol, and that alcoholism abuse and alcohol dependence may mask an underlying affective illness. Women, on the other hand, more frequently manifest depressive or dysphoric symptoms with less coexistence of alcoholism, and are thus diagnosed as psychiatrically ill earlier in the course of their affective illness.

An association between bipolar illness and alcoholism has also gained increasing attention (Winokur et al., 1969). A number of clinical trials with lithium are underway for alcoholic patients as well as for alcoholic patients with coexistent affective illness (Goodwin et al., 1969).

The standardized diagnostic approaches used with samples of patients in treatment for alcoholism indicate a considerable co-morbidity of alcohol problems and other mental disorders. Attention has been drawn to the coexistence of not only alcoholism and affective disorders, but also to the coexistence of alcohol dependence or abuse with anxiety disorders and antisocial personality.

Several risk factors associated with alcoholism have received attention from social psychiatric and interpersonal schools. In addition to the sex differences previously noted, the role of intrafamilial dynamics in early childhood and in adulthood has been emphasized. Numerous cultural and psychosocial factors have also been identified to explain the observed differences in prevalence of alcoholism among various ethnic groups. The influence of social and cultural values and family interaction patterns have been investigated to account for variations in rates among different ethnic groups.

The interpersonal school has drawn attention to the role of intrafamilial dynamics in perpetuating alcoholic behavior. The special burden of the illness on spouses of alcoholics, particularly wives, and on children have been the focus of concern in the alcoholism community, particularly through Alanon.

The behavioral school has been mainly involved in the development of therapeutic interventions based upon conditioning paradigms. The use of antabuse and aversive conditioning with drugs, such as Emetine, represent a combination of pharmacologic and conditioning approaches to treatment.

Drug Abuse

Concern for the adverse psychiatric consequences of drugs emerged in the U.S. during the mid 19th century after the Civil War. Two developments contributed to that concern: the innovation of the hypodermic syringe and the introduction of morphine.

By the end of the 19th century, the clinical features of addiction were identified: increasing dose requirements, psychological craving and dependence, and withdrawal syndrome upon cessation of use. Public concern over the adverse effects of the opiates and other narcotics resulted in the enactment of the Harrison Act in 1908. Soon afterward, there was widespread debate about heroin and other opium derivatives. The U.S. Public Health Service developed a research unit for addiction in Lexington, Kentucky, after World War II, which undertook major research on the pharmacology of narcotic drugs and the clinical manifestations of their use. This unit is now located in Baltimore, Maryland.

Between World Wars I and II, interest extended to other classes of drugs, including marijuana, barbiturates and amphetamines. Concern accelerated after World War II over the rapid expansion of the use of heroin, amphetamines and marijuana as well as the new synthetic hallucinogens, LSD and PCP. These concerns were reflected in increasing scientific research, the creation by Congress of the National Institute on Drug Abuse (NIDA), and controversy surrounding the social, legal and treatment aspects of drug abuse. The "amotivational syndrome" described by a number of clinicians has not been completely validated and remains another source of controversy.

This section has reviewed the current state of research and theory in selected diagnostic groups. For each disorder, the approach to diagnosis and related research activities has been discussed in terms of the foci of the major schools. The framework for discussion has been predominantly, but not exclusively, the classification embodied in DSM-III.

VI. Conclusions

Heinz Lehmann's observation in 1970 that North American psychiatry was on the verge of a revival of interest in diagnosis has proven prophetic. The 1970s witnessed a series of major developments in clinical psychopathology leading to the reaffirmation of the concepts of discrete disorders and of the importance for research, training and clinical practice of reliable and well-validated criteria for diagnosis and classification.

The current period is one of considerable activity in the area of diagnosis and classification in relation to psychopathology. Operational criteria, improved techniques for developing reliability and clarification of the nature of validity, which were crystallized in the development of the DSM-III, have diffused rapidly throughout the research community and into the clinical community as well.

The schools of American psychiatry have reacted to these developments with varying degrees of involvement. The greatest acceptance has been by the biological school because of the application of these concepts toward understanding the actions of the new psychopharmacologic agents. The social psychiatry school has rapidly incorporated these diagnostic techniques in new and important epidemiologic studies attempting to determine the incidence and prevalence of psychiatric disorders, as well as to ascertain psychosocial, familial and biological risk factors. These new techniques and concepts slowly are being incorporated in behavioral, interpersonal and psychoanalytical research and practice.

Agreement is widespread concerning the heuristic value of defining clinical syndromes on the basis of descriptive psychopathological criteria. At the same time, dissatisfaction exists regarding exclusive reliance on the symptomatic approach to diagnosis. Most investigators share the ideal of validating diagnosis by etiology. This aim is most evident in the search for biological factors which may be etiologic, but is also seen in the search for behavioral, childhood experience, personality and other nonbiological antecedents. It is now widely recognized, however, that in the past premature closure on presumed etiological factors contributed to confusion and unreliability.

While there is recognition that the availability of operational criteria has improved reliability and clarified many problems, a number of issues remain unresolved. These include the overlap between affective states and schizophrenia, including the unsettled status of schizo-affective states; the best manner in which to subdivide affective disorders; and the cross-diagnosis of alcoholism and drug abuse, on the one hand, and, on the other hand, the diagnostic relation between alcoholism and/or drug abuse and other psychiatric syndromes. In the areas of clinical care and research, efforts are underway to find laboratory and other nonclinical procedures to supplement clinical diagnostic criteria.

The most difficult problems, however, are with the personality disorders and developmental states included in Axis II, where the research challenge is to clarify the relationship between dimensional and typological approaches. Still unsettled is the basic issue of whether personality disorders represent discrete categories defined by typological criterion, or, rather, points of distribution on dimensional criteria. Considerable efforts are underway in this area, particularly research to validate disorders such as narcissistic and borderline personality disorders, as well as traditional personality disorders that have been fully validated, such as passive-aggressive personality disorder.

Even with these unsolved problems, efforts in the United States focused on issues of psychiatric diagnosis, nosology and classification evince considerable theoretical and conceptual ferment and a high level of research activity. There is an air of optimism and hope that new and developing approaches in the field will contribute to resolving issues of long-standing uncertainty and controversy.

VII. References

Abraham K. *Selected papers of Karl Abraham*. London: Hogarth Press, 1927.

Akiskal H, Bitar A, Puzantian V, Rosenthal T, Walker P. The nosological studies of neurotic depression. *Arch Gen Psychiatry* 35: 756, 1978.

American Psychiatric Association. *Diagnostic and statistical manual of mental disorders* (3rd edition) (DSM-III). Washington, DC: Author, 1980.

American Psychiatric Association. *Diagnostic and statistical manual of mental disorders* (Revised edition) (DSM-III-R). Washington, DC: Author, 1987.

Armor D, Klerman GL. Psychiatric treatment orientations and professional ideology. *J Health and Soc Behav* 9: 243, 1968.

Barlow DH, DiNardo PA, Vermilyea BB, Vermilyea J, Blanchard EB. Co-morbidity and depression among anxiety disorders: Issues in diagnosis and classification. *J Nerv and Ment Dis* 174: 63–72, 1986.

Beard G. *Practical treaties on nervous exhaustion (neurasthenia)*. New York: William Wood, 1880.

Beck A. Measuring depression: The depression inventory. In: Williams TA, Katz MM, Shield JA. (Eds) *Proceedings of the NIMH workshop and recent advances in the psychology of depressive illnesses*. Washington, DC: U.S. Government Printing Office, 1969.

Bockoven JS. *Moral treatment in American psychiatry*. New York: Springer Publishing Co., 1963.

Cattell RB. *Personality and motivation structure and measurement*. New York: Harcourt Brace and World, 1957.

Derogatis L, Lipman R, Covi L. SCL-90: An outpatient psychiatric rating scale: Preliminary report. *Psychopharm Bull* 9: 13, 1973.

Durkheim E. *Suicide*. New York: The Free Press, 1951.

Erikson E. *Identity: Youth and crisis*. New York: Norton, 1968.

Faris RE, Dunham H. *Mental disorders in urban areas: An ecological study of schizophrenia and other psychoses*. Chicago: University of Chicago Press, 1939.

Feighner J, Robins E, Guze S et al. Diagnostic criteria for use in psychiatric research. *Arch Gen Psychiatry* 26: 57, 1972.

Fenichel O. *The psychoanalytical theory of neurosis*. New York: Norton, 1945.

Fleiss JL, Spitzer RL, Endicott J, Cohen JL. Quantification of agreement in multiple psychiatric diagnosis. *Arch Gen Psychiatry* 26: 168, 1972

Foucault M. *Madness and civilization: A history of insanity in the age of reason*. New York: Norton, Pantheon Books, 1965.

Frances, A. The DSM-III personality disorders section: A commentary. *Am J Psychiatry* 137: 1050, 1980.

Glass A. Principles of combat psychiatry. *Military Med* 117: 27, 1955.

Goldhammer H, Marshall A. *Psychosis and civilization: Two studies in the frequency of mental disease*. New York: The Free Press, 1953.

Goodwin D. *Is alcoholism hereditary?* New York: Oxford University Press, 1976.

Goodwin FK, Murphy DL, Bunney WE, Jr. Lithium carbonate treatment in depression and mania: A longitudinal double-blind study. *Arch Gen Psychiatry* 21: 486, 1969.

Grinker R. The borderline syndrome: A phenomenological view. In: Hartocollis P. (Ed) *Borderline personality disorders*. New York: International Universities Press, 1977.

Grinker R, Spiegel J. *Men under stress*. New York: McGraw-Hill, 1945.

Grob G. *Mental institutions in America: Social policy to 1875*. New York: The Free Press, 1973.

Gruenberg E. Evaluating the effectiveness of community mental health services. *Milbank Memorial Fund Quarterly*. Part II, January, 1966.

Gunderson J, Singer M. Defining borderline patients: An overview. *Am J Psychiatry* 132: 1, 1975.

Guze S. The need for toughmindedness in psychiatric thinking. *Southern Medical Journal* 63: 662, 1970.

Guze S, Woodruff R, Clayton P. Sex, age, and the diagnosis of hysteria (Briquet's syndrome). *Am J Psychiatry* 129: 121, 1972.

Hale N. *Freud and the Americans*. New York: Oxford University Press, 1971.

Hamilton M. A rating scale for depression. *J Neurol Neurosurg Psychiat* 23: 56, 1960.

Havens L. *Approaches to the mind*. Boston: Little, Brown and Company, 1973.

Hirschfeld R. Paper presented at the World Psychiatric Association. London: 1980.

Hollingshead A, Redlich F. *Social class and mental illness*. New York: John Wiley and Company, 1958.

Holmes T, Rahe R. The social readjustment rating scale. *J Psychosomatic Res* 2: 213, 1967.

Illich I. *Medical nemesis: The expropriation of health*. London: Pantheon Books, 1976.

Joint Commission on Mental Illness and Health. *Action for mental health*. New York: Basic Books, 1961.

Katz M, Klerman GL. Introduction: Overview of the Clinical Studies Program. *Am J Psychiatry* 136: 49, 1979.

Kety SS, Rosenthal D, Wender P et al. The types and prevalence of mental illness in the biological and adoptive families of adopted schizophrenics. In: Rosenthal D, Kety SS. (Eds) *The transmission of schizophrenia*. Oxford, England: Pergamon Press, 1968.

Kiloh L, Garside R. The independence of neurotic depression and endogenous depression. *Br J Psychiatry* 109: 451, 1963.

Klerman GL, Barrett JE. The affective disorders: Clinical and epidemiological aspects. In: Gershon S, Shopsin B. (Eds) *Lithium: Its role in psychiatric treatment and research*. New York: Plenum Press, 1973.

Klerman GL. Mental illness, the medical model and psychiatry. *J Medicine and Philosophy* 2: 220, 1977.

Klerman GL. *The neo-Kraepelinian revival in American psychiatry: Its history, promise and prospect*. Presented at Scientific Symposium honoring Dr. Eli Robins; by the Department of Psychiatry, Washington University School of Medicine, St. Louis, Missouri, May 27, 1977.

Klerman GL. The psychobiology of affective states: The legacy of Adolph Meyer. In: Brady J, Meyer E. (Eds) *Psychobiology of human behavior*. Baltimore: Johns Hopkins University Press, 1979.

Klerman GL, Endicott J, Spitzer R, Hirschfeld RMS. Neurotic depression. *Am J Psychiatry* 136: 57, 1979.

Knight R. Borderline states. *Bulletin of the Menninger Clinic* 17: 1, 1953.

Kohut H. Forms and transformations of narcissism. *J Am Psychoanalytic Assoc* 14: 243, 1966.

Kohut H. *The analysis of the self*. New York: International Universities Press, 1971.

Kraepelin E. *Dementia praecox paraphrenia*. (1919) Robertson GM (Ed). Huntington, NY: Krieger, 1971.

Kramer M. Cross-national study of diagnosis of the mental disorders: Origin of the problem. *Am J Psychiatry* 125: 1, 1969.

Krauthammer C, Klerman GL. Secondary mania: Manic syndromes associated with antecedent physical illness. *Arch Gen Psychiatry* 35: 1333, 1978.

Kuhn R. The treatment of depression states with G2235 (imipramine hydrochloride). *Am J Psychiatry* 115: Nov. 1958.

Laing RD. *Laing and anti-psychiatry*. Boyers R. (Ed). New York: Harper and Row, 1971.

Lazare A. (Ed) *Outpatient psychiatry*. London: Williams and Wilkins, 1979.

Leighton D, Harding J et al. Psychiatric findings of the Stirling County Study. *Am J Psychiatry* 119: 1021, 1963.

Lemert E. *Human deviance, social problems, and social control*. 2nd edition. Englewood Cliffs, NJ: Prentice-Hall, 1972.

London P. Ethical problems in behavior control. In: Hunt WA. (Ed) *Human behavior and its control*. Cambridge, MA, 1971.

Lorr M et al. *Inpatient Multidimensional Psychiatric Scale (IMPS)*. California: Consulting Psychiatrist Press, 1962.

Mannheim K. *Ideology and utopia*. New York: Harcourt Brace & Co., 1936.

Mayer-Gross W, Slater E, Roth M. *Clinical psychiatry*. Baltimore, MD: Williams and Wilkins, 1954.

McNair D, et al. *Profile of mood states*. California: Educational and Industrial Testing Services, 1971.

Mendels J, Cochrane C. The nosology of depression: The endogenous reactive concept. *Am J Psychiatry* 124: 1, 1968.

Meyer A. *The collected papers of Adolf Meyer. Volumes 1–4*. Winters EE. (Ed). Baltimore: Johns Hopkins University Press, 1950–1952.

Mezzich J. Multiaxial diagnostic systems in psychiatry. In: Kaplan HI, Freedman AM, Sadock BJ. (Eds) *Comprehensive textbook of psychiatry/III. Volume 1*. Baltimore: Williams and Wilkins, 1980.

Mitchell SW. Address before the fiftieth annual meeting. *J Nerv and Men Disorders* 21: 413, 1894.

Murphy J. Psychiatric labeling in cross-cultural perspective. *Science* 191: 1019, 1976.

Murray H. *Thematic Aperception Test manual*. Cambridge, MA: Harvard University Press, 1953.

Musto D. *The American disease origins of narcotic control*. New Haven: Yale University Press, 1973.

Overall J, Gorham D. Brief Psychiatric Rating Scale. *Psychol Reports* 10: 799, 1962.

Perry JC, Klerman GL. The borderline patient: A comparative analysis of four sets of diagnostic criteria. *Arch Gen Psychiatry* 38: 10, 1978.

Robins E. New concepts in the diagnosis of psychiatric disorders. *Annual Review of Med* 28: 67, 1977.

Robins L. The development and characteristics of the NIMH Diagnostic Interview Schedule. In: Weissman MM, Meyers J, Ross C. (Eds) *Epidemiologic community surveys*. New York: Neale Watson Academic Publisher, 1981.

Robins E, Guze S. Establishment of psychiatric validity in psychiatric illness: Its application to schizophrenia. *Am J Psychiatry* 126: 983, 1970.

Robins E, Guze S. Classification of affective disorders. In: Williams TA, Katz MM, Shield JA. (Eds) *Recent advances in the psychobiology of depressive illness: The primary-secondary, the endogenous-reactive and the neurotic-psychotic concepts*. Washington, DC: U.S. Government Printing Office, 1972.

Rosenham D. On being sane in insane places. *Science* 197: 250, 1973.

Roth M, Argyle N. Anxiety, panic and phobic disorders: An overview. *J Psychiatric Res* 22: Supplement 1, 33–54, 1988.

Rothman D. *The discovery of the asylum: Social order and disorder in the new republic*. Boston: Little, Brown and Co., 1971.

Rothman D. *Conscience and convenience: The asylum and its alternatives in progressive America*. Boston: Little, Brown and Co., 1980.

Scheff T. *Being mentally ill: A sociological theory*. Chicago: Aldine, 1966.

Scheff T. *Labeling madness*. Englewood Cliffs, NJ: Prentice-Hall, 1975.

Skodal AE, Spitzer RL. DSM-III: Rationale, basic concepts and some differences from ICD-9. *Acta Psychiatr Scand* 66: 271–281, 1982.

Spitzer RL, Endicott J. Medical and mental disorders: Proposed definitions and criteria. In: Spitzer RL, Klein DF. (Eds) *Critical issues in psychiatric diagnosis*. New York: Raven Press, 1978.

Spitzer RL, Endicott J, Robins E. *Research diagnostic criteria (RDC) for a selected group of functional disorders*. New York State Department of Mental Hygiene, Biometrics Branch, 1975.

Srole L, Fischer A. The midtown-Manhattan longitudinal study vs the mental illness paradise lost doctrine. *Arch Gen Psychiatry* 37: 209, 1980.

Stouffer S. *Measurement and prediction*. New York: John Wiley and Sons, 1950.

Strauss A, Schatzman L et al. *Psychiatric ideologies and institutes*. New York: The Free Press, 1964.

Szasz T. *The myth of mental illness*. New York: Harper-Hoeber, 1961; Harper & Row, 1974.

Vaillant G, Perry JC. Personality disorders. In: Kaplan H, Freedman J, Sadock J. (Eds) *Comprehensive textbook of psychiatry/III*. 3rd edition. Baltimore: Williams and Wilkins, 1980.

Weissman MM, Klerman GL. Epidemiology of mental disorders. *Arch Gen Psychiatry* 35: 705, 1978.

Wing J, Cooper J et al. *The measurement and classification of psychiatric symptoms.* London: Cambridge University Press, 1974.

Winokur G, Clayton P, Reich T. *Manic-depressive disease.* St. Louis: Mosby, 1969.

Winokur G, Reich T et al. Alcoholism, III: Diagnosis and familial psychiatric illness in 259 alcoholic probands. *Arch Gen Psychiatry* 23: 104, 1970.

World Health Organization. *International classification of diseases.* 9th Edition. Washington, DC: World Health Organization, 1980.

World Health Organization. *Report of the International Pilot Study of Schizophrenia. Volume 2.* Washington, DC: World Health Organization, 1978.

Zubin J. Cross-national study of diagnosis of the mental disorders: Methodology and planning. *Am J Psychiatry* 125: 12, 1969.

Zung W. A self-rating depression scale. *Arch Gen Psychiatry* 12: 63, 1965.

5

A Brief History of Psychiatric Classification in Britain

R. E. Kendell*

Historical Background

17th and 18th Centuries

The historical origins of the diagnostic concepts of British psychiatrists are difficult to define with any clarity. They are woven into the history and prehistory of psychiatry and have much in common with those of the French and German schools, particularly with the former. Although classifications of disease in which different varieties of madness figured prominently were developed in the 17th century by Robert Burton and Thomas Willis, both were essentially Galenical, and in neither case does the author's reputation rest on the classification or the diagnostic concepts they introduced. The first, and perhaps the only, British classification to achieve worldwide influence was that of the Edinburgh physician William Cullen. His *Synopsis and Nosology*, published in 1769, was an elaborate and grandiose attempt to classify illness according to the Linnaean principle of classes, orders, genera and species. It is to him that we owe the term neurosis, introduced as a generic title for all mental disorders. Cullen assigned the second class of his classification to these neuroses, subdivided into 4 orders, 27 genera and over 100 species, and including a large group of "vesaniae," paranoid illnesses he described in detail in a later book, *First Lines of the Practice of Physik*. His classification owed its inspiration and much of its reputation to the earlier work of the botanist physicians, Boissier de Sauvages and Carl von Linné, and it was not long before its complexity and pretentions provoked a sceptical reaction. In 1782, Thomas Arnold poured scorn on Cullen and his fellow "botanical nosologists" and insisted that there

---

* University Department of Psychiatry, Royal Edinburgh Hospital, Edinburgh, Scotland, UK.

was only one genus of mental illness, that of insanity, and only two forms of insanity, ideal and notional.

19th Century

The conflict between complexity and simplicity exemplified by this dispute persisted throughout the 19th century largely because, in the absence of any agreed corpus of knowledge about the causes of madness or any specific treatments, the matter was not susceptible to resolution. One man's opinion was as good as another's, and as a result many asylums had private classifications of their own, reflecting the personal views of the physician superintendent. David Skae, for example, recognized 27 varieties of insanity, mostly of his own invention. His classification was used by a number of his friends and pupils, but when Clouston, his successor at the Edinburgh Royal Asylum, urged its more general adoption, it was rejected out of hand by Crichton Browne (Chrichton Browne, 1875) as being "philosophically unsound, scientifically inaccurate and practically useless."

Throughout the 19th century, most theoretical or conceptual—as opposed to administrative or therapeutic—innovations were derived from French or German writers: Pinel, Esquirol and Heinroth in the first half of the century; Wernicke, Morel and Charcot in the second. The one important diagnostic concept to be introduced by a British alienist in that era was Prichard's moral insanity—"a morbid perversion of the feelings, affections and active powers, without any illusion or erroneous conviction impressed upon the understanding," which "sometimes coexists with an unimpaired state of the intellectual faculties" (Prichard, 1835). This novel extension of the boundaries of insanity led to the now defunct legal concepts of the moral imbecile (1913) and moral defective (1927), and ultimately to the concept of the antisocial psychopath.

If British psychiatry had a distinctive theoretical orientation at this time it was one of pragmatism, reflecting the managerial needs and attitudes of the asylum officers of the day. In the main their preference was for simple groupings based on symptoms, course and other readily observable phenomena, and they tended to distrust elaboration and complexity, particularly elaborate classifications based on exciting but unproven speculations about etiology. It was the fanciful etiological assumptions on which it was based that made Skae's classification unacceptable to Crichton Browne. Although he accepted the ultimate desirability of an etiological classification he was convinced the time was not yet ripe. "We are still as far as ever from mounting a delusion in Canada balsam, or from detecting despondency in a test-tube," he remarked, and that being so, the simple behavioural classification of Esquirol was preferable to more elaborate and pretentious alternatives (Crichton Browne, 1875). This attitude was shared by Henry Maudsley, the dominant intellect of the day. In the 3rd edition of his *Pathology of Mind* (1879), he defended his preference for a simple symptom-based classification as follows:

> This necessity of calling up by a general term the conception of a certain co-existence and sequence of symptoms is a reason why the old classification holds its ground against classifications that are alleged to be more scientific; it is good as far as it goes, but it by no means goes to the root of the matter; whereas the classifications which pretend to go to the root of the matter go beyond what knowledge warrants and are radically faulty.

In the 1895 edition he was even more explicit:

> I have purposely avoided mention of the numerous and elaborate classifications which, in almost distracting succession, have been formally proposed as exhaustive and tacitly condemned as useless. For the same reason I have shunned the use of the many learned names—of Greek, Latin and GraecoLatin derivation—which have been invented in appalling numbers often to denote simple things and sometimes, it may be feared, with the effect of confounding apprehension of them. Insanities are not really so different from sanities that they need a new and a special language to describe them; nor are they so separated from other nervous disorders by lines of demarcation as to render it wise to distinguish every feature of them by a special technical nomenclature.

The first attempt to introduce a uniform classification of mental disorders throughout the country was made by the Statistical Committee of the Royal Medico-Psychological Association in 1881 (Statistical Committee of the Medico-Psychological Association, 1882). It was a simple classification consisting of congenital mental deficiency (with or without epilepsy), acquired epilepsy, general paralysis of the insane, four types of dementia, five of melancholia and six of mania. Its authors expressed the modest hope that even if "some Superintendents will prefer not to follow the subclasses it is hoped that all will be willing to adopt the primary classes, and that uniformity of classification will to this extent be attained." They were quickly disillusioned. Despite the efforts of their energetic and influential chairman, Hack Tuke, and a series of revisions in 1904, 1905 and 1906, most of the Association's members continued to use their own private classifications, and the attempt to achieve uniformity was finally abandoned when the radically new concepts introduced by Kraepelin and Bleuler threw everything into a state of flux. An almost identical sequence of events took place in the United States of America.

1900—1950

For the first three decades of the 20th century there were few theoretical developments of any importance in British psychiatry. Kraepelin's concepts of manic-depressive insanity and dementia praecox were accepted fairly quickly, and the prestige of the German university clinics increased steadily. But although Bleuler's term, schizophrenia, eventually displaced Kraepelin's dementia praecox, his etiological assumptions never became so influential as they did in North America. The same was true of the influence of the Viennese school of psychoanalysis. Although Freud's writings were well known and much discussed, the psychoanalytic movement never developed the widespread influence on British psychiatry that it had in the USA in the 1940s and 1950s. Psychoanalytic clinics flourished in London, particularly after the arrival of Freud himself and his daughter Anna, but they never became a dominant influence within the walls of the mental hospitals or in the new university departments of psychiatry. And despite an increasingly close political relationship with France contact with French ideas was lost almost completely after Janet's day.

A more distinctive British school of psychiatry, and with it a distinctive attitude to classification, began to emerge in the 1930s. The Maudsley Hospital, the embodiment of Henry Maudsley's vision of a university psychiatric clinic on the German model, had opened in 1919, and the University of Edinburgh had established a chair of psychiatry in the same year. Other small university departments of psychiatry started to be created from that time on. These embryonic departments were greatly strengthened by an influx of distinguished German and Austrian refugees in the late 1930s, notably Mayer Gross and Guttman from Heidelberg and Stengel from Vienna. Another crucial influence was that of Adolph Meyer, for several of the most influential teachers of that generation, including Aubrey Lewis at the Maudsley Hospital and David Henderson in Edinburgh, had been his pupils in Baltimore and had brought his distinctive holistic views back to Europe with them. These, then, were the predominant influences as British psychiatry began to expand its influence after the Second World War—the German academic tradition, particularly that of the Heidelberg school; a distrust of elaborate theoretical formulations inherited from Henry Maudsley and other 19th century alienists, and Adolph Meyer. To these were added the scholarship, skepticism and emphasis on empirical evidence of Aubrey Lewis and the new Institute of Psychiatry at the Maudsley hospital. The experience of treating and rehabilitating the psychiatric casualties of war, the psychoanalytic movement and changing public attitudes to mental illness were other important influences, but their main effect was on the milieu of mental hospitals and the development of new social and psychological forms of treatment rather than on diagnostic concepts and attitudes to classification.

After the abandonment of the Royal Medico-Psychological Association's attempt to introduce a uniform national classification at the end of the 19th century, the main influence on diagnostic concepts was exerted by influential teachers, particularly through their textbooks. In the 1940s and 1950s Henderson and Gillespie's textbook was pre-eminent, and as a result the concept of involutional melancholia and Henderson's rather muddled ideas on psychopathy both gained wide currency. The publication of Mayer Gross' textbook in 1954, however, resulted in a new emphasis on the importance of diagnostic distinctions between endogenous and reactive illnesses, and on the constitutional and genetic rather than the psychological and social determinants of psychiatric illness.

British Psychiatry and the International Classification

Soon after its formal creation in 1948, the WHO produced a 6th revision of the International Statistical Classification of Diseases, Injuries and Causes of Death. This was more important than it sounds because previous editions had been concerned only with causes of death, whereas this 1948 revision was for the first time a comprehensive nosology covering the whole range of disease—and so included a classification of mental illness. In fact, Section V of ICD-6, entitled Mental, Psychoneurotic and Personality Disorders, contained 10 categories of psychosis, 9 of psychoneurosis and 7 of "disorders of character, behaviour and intelligence," most of them subdivided further. This classification was adopted for official use in the United Kingdom, and since that time the successive editions of the International Classification have been used by the Ministry of Health and its successor, the Department of Health and Social Security, in all official documents and in its statistical analyses of admissions to mental hospitals and other psychiatric inpatient units. This is not to say, however, that either ICD-6 or its successors have been widely used by British psychiatrists. Whether or not they were even aware of the existence of the International Classification, and in the 1950s many were not, most psychiatrists continued to use whatever diagnostic terms they thought fit, and the clerks and statisticians engaged in the compilation of statistical returns had to convert these into the official nomenclature as best they could.

Unsatisfactory as this state of affairs was, from the point of view of the WHO it was less serious than that in most other countries. Although the nomenclature of ICD-6 had been unanimously adopted by the 1948 revision conference and duly "recommended for use" by all Member States, only five countries had ever adopted the Mental Disorders section of the classification, the others being Finland, New Zealand, Peru and Thailand.

In 1958, the WHO asked Erwin Stengel to investigate the situation worldwide and if possible to make recommendations. His report is an impressive document (Stengel, 1959). The situation he encountered he described as one of "almost general dissatisfaction with the state of psychiatric classification, national and international," and the attitude of many psychiatrists toward classification, at least in its conventional forms, seemed to have become "one of ambivalence, if not cynicism." Stengel was convinced that the most important reason for the inability, or refusal, of psychiatrists to agree to use a common nomenclature, national or international, lay in the etiological implications of diagnostic terms, and that it was the objections of different schools of psychiatry to each other's assumptions about etiology that lay at the root of the problem. His answer to this problem, and his most important recommendation, was that all diagnoses should be explicitly shorn of their etiological implications and regarded simply as "operational definitions" for certain specified types of abnormal behaviour. He also recommended that in future revisions of the International Classification the nomenclature should be accompanied by a companion glossary "available from the beginning in as many languages as possible."

Spurred on by this report and the chaotic situation it revealed, the WHO and its Expert Committee on Mental Health made strenuous efforts to improve the Mental Disorders Section of the International Classification, to persuade more countries to use it and to provide a companion glossary that would facilitate its use. When it became apparent that it was going to take too long to secure agreement on the wording of an international glossary, it was decided as an interim measure to encourage individual countries to produce their own national glossaries to the nomenclature of the 8th revision. The United Kingdom responded to this invitation, as did the American Psychiatric Association, and a committee set up by the Registrar General under the chairmanship of Sir Aubrey Lewis produced a UK glossary in time for the introduction of ICD-8 (General Register Office, 1968). For the next decade this booklet had a valuable but limited role. It provided some useful guidance on the meaning and scope of the various categories of disorder recognized in ICD-8, and experience of its use paved the way for the production some years later of the International Glossary (WHO, 1974). Indeed, as Lewis was chairman of the WHO working Group responsible for this and several other British psychiatrists were also involved, several sections of the International Glossary were derived from the UK glossary. Nevertheless, this British glossary had serious limitations. In the first place, it had the inevitable shortcomings of any purely national glossary. Some categories, like latent schizophrenia, were defined in completely different ways from the other (American) national glossary to ICD-8, and the reactive psychoses introduced into ICD-8 at the urging of Norwegian and Danish psychiatrists were described in terms that amounted to an invitation to ignore them. Secondly, and more fundamentally, none of the glossary's definitions were the operational definitions Stengel had advocated. They were thumbnail sketches describing the core of the concept in question tolerably well, but they gave little guidance on where its boundaries lay or what minimum criteria had to be met before the diagnosis was made. But perhaps most important of all, the glossary had little impact on the diagnostic practice of the majority of British psychiatrists. Although it was used by several groups for research purposes, a comparison of the diagnoses given to two random samples of 1000 first admissions to English mental hospitals in1968 and 1971, i.e., before and after the introduction of the new nomenclature of ICD-8 and its companion glossary, revealed no detectable difference between the two (Kendell, 1973). In both, over one-third of all diagnoses could not be converted into any category at all in either ICD-6 or ICD-8, and the many new terms introduced in the latter, such as transient situational disturbance and reactive psychosis, were still conspicuously absent in 1971.

This study also shed light on the diagnostic predilections of English psychiatrists working outside the main teaching centres. It revealed the same preference for broadly based clinical syndromes and the same distrust of fine distinctions and etiological assumptions that Crichton Browne and Henry Maudsley had expressed almost a century before. Over 50% of all depressive illnesses were described simply as "Depression" or "Depressive illness." The majority of personality disorders and schizophrenic illnesses were likewise described simply as "Personality Disorder" and "Schizophrenia." Indeed, the only schizophrenic subtype to be diagnosed with any frequency was paranoid schizophrenia, and many of the classical diagnoses were remarkably rare. In the entire series of 2000 diagnoses, there were only three of melancholia and four of involutional melancholia. Even the diagnosis of manic-depressive psychosis appeared only 20 times. Similarly, in the schizophrenic domain, there were only two diagnoses of catatonic schizophrenia, three of simple schizophrenia, five of hebephrenia and none at all of paranoia. Another notable characteristic, which presumably reflected a distrust of neat diagnostic boundaries, was the presence of many "half-and-half" diagnoses like "anxiety depression" and schizoaffective disorder.

Recent British Research on Classification

It is clear from the preceding discussion that in the 19th century, and for some time thereafter, classification did not interest British psychiatrists as much as their French and German counterparts. Zilboorg's wry comment that "to produce a well-ordered classification almost seemed to have become the unspoken ambition of every psychiatrist of industry and promise" was directed mainly at continental Europe. In the 1920s, however, a controversy developed in Britain over the classification of depressive illnesses which has continued ever since. Although super- ficially this controversy was and is concerned purely with depressive illnesses, it has continued so long, and so much time and energy have been devoted to it, partly at least because it serves as a convenient arena for several broader disputes about the nature and classification of mental illness as a whole: whether mental illnesses are diseases or reaction types; whether they are independent entities or arbitrary concepts; whether they should be classified on the basis of their symptomatology, their etiology, their pathogenesis or a mixture of all three; and whether they are better portrayed by a topology or by dimensions.

The controversy was started in 1926 by Edward Mapother, the first professor of psychiatry at the Maudsley hospital, suggesting that the distinction between neurosis and psychosis was primarily a matter of administrative convenience, and that there were no fundamental differences between them. This heretical assertion led to a prolonged and at times rather acrimonious debate about the relationship between psychotic and neurotic depressions; one school, headed by Crichton Miller and later by Mayer Gross and his protegé Martin Roth, claimed that the two were distinct illnesses, differing in symptomatology, etiology and prognosis; the other, headed by Mapother and Lewis at the Maudsley Hospital, argued that "to set up a sharp distinction 'in the interests of academic accuracy' when the distinction is not found in nature is no help to thought or action" (Lewis, 1934). The development in the late 1950s of elaborate techniques of multivariate analysis and the computers necessary for their utilization shifted the argument to a more empirical and statistical plane. Various forms of factor analysis, discriminant function analysis and cluster analysis were enthusiastically and at times rather uncritically applied to ratings of the symptomatology of cohorts of depressed patients, but without any real change in the nature of the controversy, or any agreed outcome. It all led, however, to a better appreciation of the complexity of the relationship between symptomatology, life events, treatment response and long-term course, and also to a clearer understanding of the crucial need for representative samples of patients and reliable clinical ratings.

This increasing awareness of the vital importance of reliable ratings of symptomatology led to the development of structured interviewing methods. In the USA the lead was taken by Joseph Zubin's Biometrics Research Unit in New York whose *Mental Status Schedule* and its successor the *Psychiatric Status Schedule* stipulated the precise wording and the sequence of every question the patient was asked. In Britain, the initiative was taken by the Medical Research Council's Social Psychiatry Unit at the Maudsley Hospital, and that unit's interest in psychotic illness led to the development of a semi-structured interview that allowed the interviewer significantly more freedom and flexibility. The *Present State Examination* developed by John Wing and his colleagues in the late 1960s struck the right balance between rigidity and flexibility and was also sufficiently comprehensive to cover the whole range of functional illness (Wing et al., 1974). It was therefore well suited to the study of psychotic symptomatology and was soon used extensively both in Britain and further afield. Indeed, it became the main clinical instrument in the International Pilot Study of Schizophrenia and also in the US/UK Diagnostic Project. The primary purpose of the latter was to investigate the major differences—of up to 20-fold in some age groups—in hospital first-admission rates for schizophrenia and manic depressive illness between the USA and England and Wales. Representative samples of patients were examined in New York and London using the *Present State Examination* and other structured interviewing methods and the same diagnostic criteria applied to both (Cooper et al. 1972). In the event the huge differences in observed admission rates in the two countries proved to be due entirely to differences in diagnostic criteria, American psychiatrists having a much broader concept of schizophrenia than their British counterparts and a correspondingly more restricted concept of manic depressive illness. Although in a sense this was a disappointing finding, because it put an end to several interesting speculations about why schizophrenia should be commoner in America than in Britain, it did have the salutary effect of convincing all concerned of the overriding need for uniform and reliable diagnostic criteria. The project also generated a large volume of reliable clinical ratings of representative samples of psychiatric inpatients, and these ratings were used for a number of subsidiary studies—of the relationships between schizophrenic and affective psychoses and between psychotic and neurotic depressions, and of the prognostic validity of different operational definitions of schizophrenia. Members of the project team also carried out relatively small-scale studies of variation in diagnostic criteria within the British Isles; of differences in the diagnostic criteria of German, French and British psychiatrists; and of the types of information used in the decision-making process leading to a clinical diagnosis.

In the 1950s a serious interest began to be taken for the first time in the psychiatric disorders of old age, prompted of course by their increasing clinical importance. In an influential pioneer study Martin Roth showed that there were major and stable differences in prognosis between the dementias, the confusional states and the functional psychoses of the senium, thus validating these three broad diagnostic categories (Roth, 1955). Other work by Roth and Felix Post explored the relationships between the paranoid illnesses of old age and paranoid schizophrenia, between cerebral arteriosclerosis and depression, and between the depressions of old and middle age. Among other things this led to general agreement that involutional melancholia was not the discrete entity an earlier generation had thought it to be, and that mild intellectual impairment in an elderly person with depressive symptoms did not necessarily predict progressive dementia.

At the other end of the scale, the emerging specialty of child psychiatry was attempting to develop a classification of childhood disorders. A WHO working party in 1967 agreed to experiment with a novel triaxial classification, and Rutter subsequently organized a formal comparison of this new multiaxial classification and the existing ICD-8 groupings. (Rutter et al., 1975). Although the reliability of ratings on its psychosocial stress axis was low, this new multiaxial classification proved superior to the uniaxial format of ICD-8 in most other respects. The clinical syndromes it recognized were more appropriate, it was better at handling psychiatric disorders associated with mental retardation and physical illness, and it was preferred by the clinicians participating in the study.

Conclusion

In summary, although British psychiatrists took less interest in classification than their French and German counterparts in the 19th century, they have taken a steadily increasing interest from the 1930s onwards. This culminated in some substantial and productive research in the 1960s and early 1970s. Since that time, however, interest in classification has tended to wane, in contrast to the USA. This is partly because research funds are now less freely available, but partly also because classification is no longer seen as an exciting and potentially rewarding area for research. The main lessons of the 1970s—the need for structured interviewing methods and the importance of operational criteria for diagnostic and other technical terms—have been well learnt, but the main focus of interest has now shifted to a new series of attempts to unravel the biological and social factors involved in the etiology of psychiatric disorders.

British psychiatry does not have, and indeed never has had, any important diagnostic concepts of its own in the way that French, American and Scandinavian psychiatry still do. There are several reasons for this. The United Kingdom has been committed to using the International Classification for longer than most other countries. Moreover, several British psychiatrists have played a prominent role in the discussions that have preceded the introduction of the last three revisions of the ICD and have often acted as consultants to the WHO. As a result, the format of the ICD has been influenced in many ways by our views and prejudices. On the other hand, our most important national prejudice—a preference for a simple classification based on a small number of major syndromes—has been consistently thwarted by the need of the WHO to secure the agreement of as many countries as possible to the nomenclature of the ICD. Because it is always more important to individual national representatives to ensure the inclusion of their own familiar diagnostic categories than it is to exclude other terms they do not wish to use, any international nomenclature has an innate tendency to expand. This is well exemplified by the variety of depressive illnesses recognized in successive revisions of the international classification. In ICD-6 and ICD-7 there were three varieties, in ICD-8 there were four and in ICD-9 there were no less than ten—even though much research in the interim had failed to validate even the primary subdivision into psychotic and neurotic depressions.

Since 1980 attitudes to classification have been dominated by the American Psychiatric Association's innovatory classification, DSM-III (APA, 1980). As in the United States there has been a clear divergence of views. The younger generation has welcomed the operational definitions, multiple axes and novel format of this nomenclature, while some of their elders have remained skeptical of the value of inflexible definitions to experienced clinicians like themselves, and have also been affronted by the elimination of hallowed terms like hysteria, neurosis and manic-depressive psychosis. Despite widespread acceptance of its basic principles, however, DSM-III has probably been used less in Britain either for research or for everyday clinical purposes than in most other English-speaking countries. This is partly because of a sense of commitment to the principle of an international classification, partly because home grown classificatory systems like Wing's CATEGO program were already available to most research workers, and partly also because earlier American criteria like the Research Diagnostic Criteria of Spitzer, Endicott and Robins (1978) seemed preferable for many purposes. It seems certain, though, that ICD-10 will be welcomed and widely used when it is finally published in 1990, even though the need to obtain the approval of psychiatrists from many divergent cultural backgrounds has already complicated the relatively simple format and nomenclature proposed by the original architects. The ICD-10 is firmly based on symptomatology, avoids premature assumptions about aetiology, recognizes the overriding importance of reliability and is therefore likely to be capable of serving as an effective international lingua franca, at least until the end of this century.

References

American Psychiatric Association (1980) *Diagnostic and Statistical Manual of Mental Disorders, 3rd Edn.* (DSM-III). Washington, D.C.: American Psychiatric Association.

Cooper, J.E., Kendell, R.E., Gurland, B.J., Sharpe, L., Copeland, J.R.M. and Simon, R. (1972) *Psychiatric Diagnosis in New York and London.* Maudsley Monograph No. 20, London: Oxford University Press.

Crichton Browne, J. (1875) Skae's classification of mental diseases: A critique. *Journal of Mental Science, 21,* 339-365.

General Register Office (1968) *A Glossary of Mental Disorders.* Studies on Medical and Population Subjects No. 22, London: HMSO.

Kendell, R.E. (1973) The influence of the 1968 glossary on the diagnoses of English psychiatrists. *British Journal of Psychiatry, 123,* 527–530.

Lewis, A.J. (1934) Melancholia: a clinical survey of depressive states. *Journal of Mental Science, 80,* 359–374.

Maudsley, H. (1879) *Physiology and Pathology of Mind. 3rd Ed.*

Prichard, J.C. (1835) *Treatise on Insanity and other Disorders Affecting the Mind.* London: Sherwood, Gilbert and Piper.

Roth, M. (1955) The natural history of mental disorder in old age. *Journal of Mental Science, 101,* 281–301.

Rutter, M., Shaffer, D. and Shepherd, M. (1975) *A Multi-Axial Classification of Child Psychiatric Disorder.* Geneva: WHO.

Spitzer, R.L., Endicott, J., Fleiss, J.L., and Cohen, J. (1970) The Psychiatric Status Schedule: A technique for evaluating psychopathology and impairment in role functioning. *Archives of General Psychiatry. 23,* 41–55.

Spitzer, R.L., Endicott, J. and Robins, E. (1978) *Research Diagnostic Criteria (RDC) for a Selected Group of Functional Disorders, 3rd edn.* New York State Psychiatric Institute.

Spitzer, R.L., Fleiss, J.L., Burdock, E.I. and Hardesty, A.S. (1964) The Mental Status Schedule: Rationale, reliability and validity. *Comprehensive Psychiatry, 5,* 384–395.

Statistical Committee of the Medico-Psychological Association (1882) Recommendations for alterations in and additions to the statistical tables of the Association. *Journal of Mental Science, 28,* 448–464.

Stengel, E. (1959) Classification of mental disorders. *Bulletin of the World Health Organization, 21,* 601–663.

Wing, J.K., Cooper, J.E. and Sartorius, N. (1974) *Description and Classification of Psychiatric Symptoms.* Cambridge: Cambridge University Press.

World Health Organization (1974) *Glossary of Mental Disorders and Guide to their Classification.* Geneva: WHO.

6

Diagnostic and Classification Tradition of Mental Disorders in the 20th Century in Scandinavia

P. Bech*

The development of the national classification systems in the Scandinavian countries in this century is shown in Table 1. In Finland, the International Classification of Diseases (ICD) was adopted in 1936 (ICD-4, ISI, 1929). Since 1952, the revisions of ICD by the World Health Organization (WHO) have been in use in Finland. The other Scandinavian countries adopted ICD-8 in 1967 upon its release (WHO, 1967). In 1987, Finland, Norway and Sweden adopted ICD-9 (WHO, 1978), whereas Denmark still uses ICD-8.

Table 1. Official classification systems of mental disorders in Scandinavia.

DENMARK	NORWAY	SWEDEN	FINLAND
Danish Psychiatric Association (1938)	Minister of Health (1894)		Institute of Medicine (1923)
			ICD-4 (ISI, 1929) from 1936
Danish Psychiatric Association (1952)	Minister of Health (1926)		
			ICD-5 (ISI, 1938)
ICD-8 (WHO, 1967)	ICD-8 (WHO, 1967)	ICD-8 (WHO, 1967)	ICD-6 (WHO, 1948) from 1952
	ICD-9 (WHO, 1978) from 1987	ICD-9 (WHO, 1978) from 1987	ICD-7 (WHO, 1955)
			ICD-8 (WHO, 1967)
			ICD-9 (WHO, 1978) from 1987

In the following, the Danish diagnostic tradition will be described in more detail. However, the diagnostic tradition in the other Scandinavian countries has been very similar to the Danish. It is of interest

---

* Department of Psychiatry, Frederiksborg General Hospital, 3400 Hillerød, Denmark.

that the first official classification system in Sweden was ICD-8, although Essen-Möller and Wohlfahrt (1947) made important suggestions for the development of a Swedish national system for classifying mental disorders. They used a multidimensional approach as had Hoche (1912) and the Swedish psychiatrist Sjöbring (1919). This approach was further developed by Essen-Möller (1971) and Ottosson and Perris (1973).

Among other Swedish studies that have had an impact on Scandinavian psychiatrists is the work of Perris (1974) on cycloid psychoses and the concept of non-regressive schizophrenia (Nyman, 1975).

As indicated in Table 1, it seems logical to discuss the period from 1938 through 1952 separately with reference to the classification system used by the Danish Psychiatric Association (DPA, 1938).

The period from 1952 through 1967 covers the use of the revised Danish classification system (DPA, 1952; Stengel, 1959), which was a two-axial system. The period from 1967 through 1987 covers the Scandinavian adoption of ICD-8, and the period since then will focus on the ICD-9 and ICD-10.

Danish Psychiatric Association 1938

The first Danish classification system of mental disorders (DPA, 1938) was based on an American system, namely, the Statistical Guide, State of New York (Committee on Forms and Statistics, 1934). Strömgren modified the American classification system in accordance with the Danish tradition (Strömgren, 1938; Borup Svendsen, 1952). For the functional psychoses, this system combined the medical model of Kraepelin (schizophrenia and manic-depressive psychoses) with the phenomenological approach of Wimmer (1916) (for psychogenic psychoses). Table 2 shows the various diagnostic systems in relation to the 15 main categories suggested by Arentsen and Strömgren (1959).

The psychogenic psychosis is one of the diagnostic categories that Danish psychiatrists have found to be important when the classification system is used for prediction of long-term course of illness and for the prediction of response to treatment. As stated by Strömgren (1974), Wimmer's monograph from 1916 represented the first comprehensive survey of the concept of psychogenic psychosis. Wimmer emphasized that psychogenic psychoses are clinically independent psychoses (from schizophrenia and manic-depressive psychosis); that they usually develop in a predisposed individual (personality deviation); and that they are caused by psychosocial factors in the sense that these factors determine the onset of the episode and the fluctuations (remissions,

SUFFICIENT EPIDEMIO-LOGICAL STATISTIC FOR MAIN DIAGNOSES (ARENTSEN & STRÖMGREN, 1959)	DANISH PSYCHIATRIC ASSOCIATION		ICD-8	ICD-8/DSM-III INTEGRATION
	1938	1952	1967	1988
1. SCHIZOPHRENIA	18	A9	295	SCHIZOPHRENIA
2. MANIC-DEPRESSIVE DISORDERS	17	A8	296	MANIC-DEPRES. PSYCHOSES
3. PRESENILE AND SENILE PSYCHOSES	11	A7	290	DEMENTIA
4. CARDIOVASCULAR DISEASE	8	A6	293	ORGANIC PSYCH.
5. NEUROSYPHILIS	1, 2	A3	292	ORGANIC PSYCH.
6. EPILEPSY	10	A10	293, 309	ORGANIC PSYCH.
7. OTHER ORGANIC DISORDERS	7, 14, 15	A3, 4, 5, 11	293, 293 294, 309	ORGANIC PSYCH.
8. PSYCHOGENIC PSYCHOSES	16,19, 20	A12	298	REACTIVE PSYCH.
9. NEUROSES	16	B	300, 305	NEUROSES
10. PSYCHOPATHIA	23, 5	C	301, 302	AXIS 2
11. MENTAL DEFICIENCY	23, 4	D	310, 315	MENTAL RETARD.
12. ALCOHOLISM	5, 6	A1	291, 303	ALCOH.USE DISOR.
13. DRUG ADDICTION	5, 6	A1	304	OTHER SUBSTAN. USE DISORDERS
14. NOT CLASSIFI-CABLE PSYCHOSES	22	A13	299	UNSPECIFIED PSYCHOSES
15. OTHER DIAGNOSES	13	A2, E, F	297,299,306 307, 308	POSSIBLE PSYCH. SYNDROME
		B	309	NON PSYCHOTIC STATE ASSOCIA-TED WITH PHYSI-CAL CONDITION
		A12	297	PARANOID STATES
			306	ANOREXIA NERV.
		F	307	ADJ. REACTION
		H	790	NO SPECIFIC PSYCH.SYNDROME

Table 2. The main diagnostic grouping by Arentsen and Strömgren (1959) compared to other systems.

intermissions, exacerbations) of the illness. Likewise, the form and content of psychosis are influenced by these psychosocial factors. Most importantly, these states have a great tendency to recover, and they seem never to end in deterioration.

The prognostic validity of psychogenic psychoses has been evaluated by Færgeman (1945, 1963), who followed up patients admitted to Wimmer's department during the years 1924 to 1926 with the diagnosis of psychogenic psychosis. The result of Færgeman's study is briefly summarized in Table 3. Of the original cases of psychogenic psychosis (N=113), 66 were later confirmed by Færgeman, whereas in 32 cases (or 28%) Faergeman made a diagnosis of schizophrenia. Of the original cases of uncertain psychogenic psychosis (N=35), 9 were later confirmed by Færgeman, 20 cases (or 57%) being diagnosed as schizophrenia. This difference is statistically significant (Table 3). However, upon reviewing Færgeman's study, Slater (1964) concluded that too many of the original cases had developed schizophrenia, which put the validity of psychogenic psychosis in serious doubt. Against this statement Strömgren (1974) has argued that the difficulties of distinguishing (in the acute state) between psychogenic psychosis and schizophrenia should lead us to sharpen our diagnostic tools rather than discard the concept of psychogenic psychosis.

FÆRGEMAN'S DIAGNOSES / WIMMER'S ORIGINAL DIAGNOSES	PSYCHOGENIC PSYCHOSES	PREDOMINANTLY SCHIZO-PHRENIA	UNCERTAIN DIAGNOSES
PSYCHOGENIC PSYCHOSES	66	32	15
UNCERTAIN PSYCHOGENIC PSYCHOSES	9	20	6

Table 3. A 16-year follow-up study of patients classified by Wimmer as suffering from psychogenic psychoses (Færgeman, 1945). The chi^2 statistic is 12.2 for the 3×2 table (2 degrees of freedom, $p \leq 0.001$), and is 10.7 for the 2×2 table excluding Færgeman's uncertain diagnosis (1 degree of freedom, $p \leq 0.001$).

The predictive value of the category of psychogenic psychosis concerning response to treatment can be analyzed from the Danish Psychiatric Association's two multi-center trials in 1938–1939. They evaluated the efficacy of insulin shock therapy (Christiansen et al., 1942) and cardiazol (pentylene tetrazol) convulsive therapy (Stürup et al., 1942). The results of these trials are shown in Table 4.

In patients with psychogenic psychoses, both cardiazol convulsive therapy and insulin shock therapy were very effective with only 22% and 15% of the non-responders, respectively (Table 4). In manic-depres-

CARDIAZOL CONVULSIVE THERAPY (STÜRUP ET AL., 1942)				INSULIN SHOCK THERAPY (CHRISTIANSEN ET AL., 1942)			
DIAGNOSIS N = 1641	IMPROVEMENT IN PERCENT			DIAGNOSIS N = 406	IMPROVEMENT IN PERCENT		
	Moderate to excellent	Slight	None or doubtful		Moderate to excellent	Slight	None or doubtful
Schizophrenia (N = 782)	5	15	80	Schizophrenia (N = 170)	8	20	72
Uncertain schizophrenia (N = 157)	27	17	56	Uncertain schizophrenia (N = 123)	34	15	51
Manic-depress. psychosis (N = 188)	59	12	29	Manic-depress. psychosis (N = 13)	23	8	69
Uncertain mnic-depress. (N = 74)	38	19	43	-	-	-	-
Psychogenic psychosis (N = 67)	63	15	22	Psychogenic psychosis (N = 19)	74	11	15
Uncertain psychogenic psychosis (N = 36)	56	16	28	Uncertain psychogenic psychosis (N = 15)	60	0	40
Depression unspecific (N = 110)	47	18	35	-	-	-	-
Uncertain diagnosis (N = 227)	46	9	45	Other or uncertain diagnosis (N = 66)	38	17	45

Table 4. The relationship between diagnoses and outcome of treatment in the two Danish multicenter trials.

sive psychosis, cardiazol convulsive therapy was found superior to insulin shock therapy with 29% versus 69% of the non-responders, respectively (χ^2 = 9.7, P<0.01). No effect was seen in schizophrenia either with cardiazol convulsive therapy nor with insulin shock therapy. These results were later confirmed in other countries, but many patients with schizophrenia had to be exposed to these treatments because the diagnostic concept of schizophrenia outside Scandinavia was too inclusive.

The narrow concept of schizophrenia in Scandinavia has also been found of high value in twin studies. Hence, when diagnosing the patients described by Gottesman and Shields (1972), Essen-Möller found a significant difference between monozygous twins (75% concordance of schizophrenia) and dizygous twins (11% concordance of schizophrenia).

The narrow concept of schizophrenia must be evaluated in relation to the concept of psychogenic paranoid psychosis. It might well be that patients with psychogenic psychosis who later develop schizophrenia have lesser biological vulnerability than patients who at the very onset of illness show pure schizophrenic manifestations.

Strömgren (1986) has summarized his experiences when discussing with colleagues from other countries the concept of psychogenic psychosis:

> . . .Whereas decades ago my lectures quite often seemed to be received with absolute lack of interest, the situation is now changing. Usually after the lecture several from the audience are asking private questions and telling me about own experiences of a similar nature, and I receive letters afterwards, but a real public discussion practically never occurs . . .

Danish Psychiatric Association 1952

In his study on psychiatric morbidity among civilians during the war using Danish psychiatric hospital admissions from 1939 to 1948, Borup Svendsen (1952) found that the DPA (1938) classification system was insufficient, because no distinction between main diagnoses and subdiagnoses was made. A multidiagnostic approach without such a distinction ". . . must be a disturbing element in reports intended for statistical purposes. At any rate, it is bound to entail a far larger number of errors than the procedure of listing only one diagnosis for each patient . . ." (Borup Svendsen, 1952).

The Danish Psychiatric Association (DPA) considered in 1952 the suggestions made by Essen-Möller and Wohlfahrt (1947) of a multidimensional system and found that this approach was too complex for the daily routine, but developed a two-compartment system. In compartment 1 the main diagnosis should be listed, and in compartment 2 the subsidiary diagnosis. The main diagnosis was defined as the condition for which admission or treatment was required. Hence, it was decided that it should be the state at the point of admission to hospital (and not the discharge diagnosis) that was the basis for the main diagnosis. A psychogenic psychosis, for instance, in a patient with psychopathic personality disorder, should be classified as psychogenic psychosis in compartment 1 and psychopathic personality disorder in compartment 2. Only one diagnosis (the most probable) should be

Table 5. Classification of the Danish Psychiatric Association 1952. In () are the corresponding numbers used in the Statistical Guide, State of New York, which was used as the first Danish classification system in 1938.

A   PSYCHOSES

    1.   INTOXICATION (05, 06)

    2.   PSYCHOTIC STATES IN GENERAL PHYSICAL DISEASES (13)

    3.   INFECTIOUS DISEASES (01, 02, 03, 04)

    4.   TRAUMATIC BRAIN LESIONS (07)

    5.   BRAIN TUMORS (14)

    6.   PSYCHOSIS WITH VASCULAR LESIONS IN THE CNS (08)

    7.   SENILE AND PRESENILE PSYCHOSES (11)

    8.   MANIC-DEPRESSIVE PSYCHOSES (17)

    9.   SCHIZOPHRENIA (18)

   10.   EPILEPSY (10)

   11.   PSYCHOSIS IN HEREDITARY ORGANIC BRAIN DISEASES (15)

   12.   PSYCHOGENIC MENTAL DISORDERS (16, 19, 20)

   13.   OTHER MENTAL DISEASES, DISEASES OF UNCERTAIN DIAGNOSES (22)

B   NEUROSES (16)

C   NON-PSYCHOTIC PERSONALITY DISORDERS

    1.   PSYCHOPHATICS (23,5   23,6)

    2.   CHARACTER NEUROSES

D   OLIGOPHRENIA (23,4)

E   OTHER DISABILITIES (E.G. DYSLEXIA)

F   ISOLATED ABNORMAL REACTIONS

    1.   AFFECTIVE REACTION

    2.   REACTION TO SHOCK

G   MENTAL ABNORMITY OF UNCERTAIN TYPE (22)

H   WITHOUT MENTAL ABNORMALITY

listed in compartment 1, but in compartment 2 more than one diagnosis was allowed, if needed. The DPA (1952) classification system is shown in Table 5 with reference to the DPA (1938) system. The DPA (1952) took reference to the relevant categories of ICD-6 (WHO, 1948), which was found to be insufficiently detailed to allow such a linkage. The DPA (1952) was used in the census study on patients in Danish psychiatric hospitals (Arentsen & Strömgren, 1959; Juel-Nielsen & Strömgren, 1963). The 15 main categories shown in Table 2 were constructed by Arentsen and Strömgren (1959), with a view toward recording sufficient statistics without losing valuable information.

Helgason (1964) used the DPA (1952) system in his outstanding analysis of the epidemiology of mental disorders in Iceland. Helgason found that the morbid risk of developing psychoses up to the age of 61 years was rather similar to the risk in the Danish population (around 1% for schizophrenia, around 2.5% for manic-depressive psychosis, and around 1% for psychogenic psychoses). The expectancy of neuroses was estimated as around 5% for males and 10% for females if only the moderate to severe cases were considered, again rather similar to the risk in the Danish population. The Danish concept of neurosis is based on the personality disorder of character neurosis (Vanggaard, 1979) for which such elements as self-perception, intrapsychic organization, striving for emotional gains and symbiotic relationship with significant other persons have to be considered.

The morbid risk of psychopathy in Helgason's study was 4% for males and 3% for females, which is rather similar to the risk in the Danish population. The Danish concept of psychopathy includes personality disorders that are distinct from psychotic personality as well as from borderline personality and from character neurosis. This personality disorder is characterized by permanent quantitative deviations that are considered pathological on the basis of a criterion of suffering of the individual or the society.

The stability of the DPA (1952) diagnoses from 1953 to 1966 has been analyzed by Marstal and Borup Svendsen (1968) using the admission rate for all mental hospitals in Denmark throughout this period. It was found that the ratio psychosis/nonpsychosis was very constant year by year (approximately 1). Within the psychotic categories the frequency of schizophrenia (around 12%), manic-depressive psychosis (around 18%) and reactive psychosis (around 12%) was also found very constant.

ICD-8

When Stengel (1959) made his inquiry into the current state of psychiatric classification systems for the revision of ICD-7 (WHO, 1955) Odegård stated: ". . . There is no room for reactive or psychogenic depressions of psychotic degree, which means that such conditions will have to be classified under manic-depressive psychosis or under neurosis . . ." (Stengel, 1959). And Strömgren added: ". . . The two main objections to ICD are that so many psychiatrically significant states are not to be found in the psychiatric part of the list, and that the terminology of neurosis differs very much from that in use in Scandinavia . . ." (Stengel, 1959).

The ICD-8 (WHO, 1967) included psychogenic or reactive psychoses and listed the mental disorders in one chapter. However, the Schneider (1958) subtyping of psychopathic personality disorders, which was included in ICD-8 and thereby gave rise to much confusion in Scandinavian statistics after ICD-8, was accepted by the various countries in 1967. The Schneider concept of psychopathy includes character neurosis and sensitive personality disorders seen in borderline cases. In this respect, the Scandinavian psychiatrists seem to follow the French-speaking psychiatrists (Pichot, 1978) in accepting at least three of Schneider's ten types, namely, the unstables or nonsyntonic dysphoria, the anempathic or social maladjustment disorder, and the abulics, who are characterized by their lack of resistance to any influence, especially a negative one (Pichot, 1978).

With the ICD-8 glossary (WHO, 1974), the guidelines for polydiagnoses (main and subsidiary diagnoses) was introduced largely following the DPA (1952) principle.

A closer look at the DPA (1952) classification (Table 5) shows the lack of categories of borderline personality disorders and schizo-affective disorders. The Scandinavian tradition of diagnosing borderline states has been influenced by Vanggaard (1955, 1979) with reference to the study of Hoch and Polatin (1949). Especially the concept of anhedonia has been used as the essential feature of borderline personality (Vanggaard, 1979), defined as a painful lack of vitality based on a narcissistic distance from other people giving rise to ontological ambivalence in interpersonal relations. Anhedonia has erroneously been associated with depression, but depressive personalities are hedonics (Bech, 1989).

As discussed by Mors (1988), the study of the use of ICD-8 in Denmark has concentrated on two categories: (1) schizophrenia, latent (code 259.59) and (2) casus limitares pseudoneurotic sive pseudopsychopathical (code 301.83). Although around 88% of Danish psychiatrists have claimed to use the concept of borderline states in their clinical work (Randløv & Parnas, 1988), results from all first admissions based on the nationwide Danish Psychiatric Register (Mors, 1988) seem to show that there are considerable variations in the geographic use of these two ICD-8 categories. Latent schizophrenia is a term that should be abandoned, because psychiatric disorders have to be classified on the basis of clinical manifestations. A psychiatric syndrome should be classified among clinical syndromes (e.g., nonregressive schizophrenia), whereas borderline states should be classified among personality disorders. Hence, both categories should be considered for each patient as suggested by Bech et al. (1987).

Within schizophrenia, the subtyping suggested by Nyman (1975), Nyman (1978) and Eberhard and Ottosson (1988) deserves particular attention. The term nonregressive schizophrenia has been suggested by these authors for pseudoneurotic schizophrenia to indicate a manifest clinical syndrome of minor schizophrenia.

Furthermore, the Scandinavian concept of schizo-affective psychosis includes varieties of manic-depressive psychoses both because of their long-term prognosis and because of their response to treatment (e.g., convulsive therapy and lithium). In ICD-8 this category is listed under schizophrenia.

The increasing use of the category of borderline cases and the trend to separate schizo-affective states from schizophrenia because of the effectiveness of lithium therapy in schizo-affective states ("atypical manic-depressive psychosis") might explain the decrease in the incidence of schizophrenia found in Danish psychiatric hospitals since 1970 (Munk-Jørgensen, 1987).

ICD-9 and ICD-10

The decision to accept ICD-9 in the Scandinavian countries (apart from Denmark) was made by colleagues in the other branches of medicine, not by psychiatrists. In Denmark, the administrative costs of changing from ICD-8 to ICD-9 were found to be too high when taking the rather small classificational benefits of ICD-9 into account.

In Finland and Norway and to some extent in Sweden, the DSM-III (APA, 1980) is being increasingly used. At a meeting comparing DSM-III and ICD-10 in November 1987 in Copenhagen, the Danish psychiatrists seemed to prefer ICD-10, although some scepticism concerning the draft version of ICD-10 was expressed. At a meeting in the WHO Collaborating Centre in Århus, February 1988, among the Danish investigators who tested the ICD-10 it was suggested to retain the concept of psychogenic or reactive psychosis as defined in ICD-8 and ICD-9; to include borderline category among personality disorders; and to create a category for mixed endogenous and reactive depression.

A modern classification system of mental disorders should be relevant for all those engaged in treatment, including general practitioners. For example, most depressed patients are now treated in general practice. The 15 main categories constructed by Arentsen and Strömgren (1959) include some categories that are infrequently seen in units in general hospital psychiatry and do not list others which are more frequent. Table 2 shows the categories that were found important in a recent study (Bech et al., 1987); these include nonpsychotic states associated with physical conditions, anorexia nervosa, adjustment reactions and unspecific psychiatric syndromes. In a study on depressed patients treated in a Danish multicenter study to evaluate a new antidepressant, it was found that around 30% of the patients had a mixture of endogenous and reactive depression (Bech et al., 1988). In this context it is of interest that the Danish neurologist Lange a century ago described mild depressive disorders in a very intensive study of about 800 outpatients whom he had treated over 12 years in his private practice. These patients were without severe neurotic features and had never developed psychotic depressions. They had presented their illness by somatic symptoms, and Lange (1896) described these patients as cases of "periodic depressions."

With the introduction of antidepressants such states of mild depression often, with somatization, were considered by Sørensen (1960) as mild endogenous depression, and these patients responded well to antidepressants. A placebo-controlled study in general practice has recently confirmed these findings (Jørgensen et al., 1984).

In a review article on somatic presentations of psychiatric illnesses in primary care setting, Goldberg and Bridges (1988) suggested that ICD-10 should include categories of uncomplicated depressive illnesses and depressive illness with somatization. This suggestion is in line with the tradition of Danish psychiatrists.

In another review article on therapeutic effects of anxiety disorders treatment, Pichot (1986) emphasizes that the Danish philosopher Kierkegaard (1844) was among the first to distinguish between normal "existential" anxiety and pathological anxiety. Odegård (1988) indicates that Kierkegaard's existential phenomenology might have influenced Wimmer when, in 1916, he described psychogenic psychosis. The so-called kayak dizziness first noticed by Lange (1864) among Eskimoes in Greenland when they were alone in their kayaks for a long period seems to be a state of agoraphobic anxiety ("nangiarnek," the Eskimo term meaning anxiety) caused by sensory deprivation (Pontoppidan, 1900). Sensory deprivation might be considered as a psychosocial stressor.

Agoraphobia is listed under the category of obsessional states in DPA (1952). However, in a comprehensive study on more than 100 patients with various forms of neuroses, Jacobsen (1965), using the DPA (1952) system, found that agoraphobia was not exclusively related to obsessional neurosis. He found that around 60% of anxiety neurotics had an agoraphobia that was as serious as that found in obsessional neurosis. Furthermore, Jacobsen found that fears of scenes with sexual and aggressive content were seen more frequently in anxiety neurosis than in obsessional neurosis. However, whereas the obsessional neurotics seemed to cope well with their drive to aggressive behavior, the anxiety neurotics suffered from the fear of being aggressive, which Jacobsen considered a phobia (eridophobia). Hence, agoraphobia and eridophobia are related to anxiety. In DSM-III phobia is included in the category of anxiety disorders.

It is essential that a classification system of mental disorders to be used by general practitioners separate pathological phobia from simple phobia and anxiety from depression. In Scandinavia this is one of the diagnostic problems that has not been solved. The hermeneutic approach of existential phenomenology and the biological approach stimulated by the development of psychopharmacological drugs have called for a multidimensional classification system. The various dimensions in such a system can then statistically consider the relevant, e.g., psychodynamic, behavioral, social or biological models (Bech, 1987).

In this century psychiatry has been separated from neurology in Scandinavia. The concept of dementia, however, is still a major link between the two. On the other hand, dementia should not be used synonymously with the concept of organic brain disorders, which is a broader concept including focal syndromes such as aphasia and amnesia. Swedish psychiatrists have recently made attempts to reconsider dementia and have found it meaningful to include both progressive and nonprogressive as well as reversible forms. The multidimensional approach seems fruitful when describing the concept of dementia and the current tradition in Sweden is shown in Figure 1 (Gottfries, 1988). The interphase between psychiatry and neurology is evident.

During the last decades clinical psychiatry has developed standardized clinical assessment methods to increase the reliability and communicational clarity when diagnosing mental disorders (e.g., Hamilton, 1967; Wing et al., 1974). These clinical methods are still considered useful tools in clinical research (e.g., WHO 1973, 1983). Scandinavian psychiatry has also been active in this field (e.g., Åsberg et al., 1978; Bech et al., 1986).

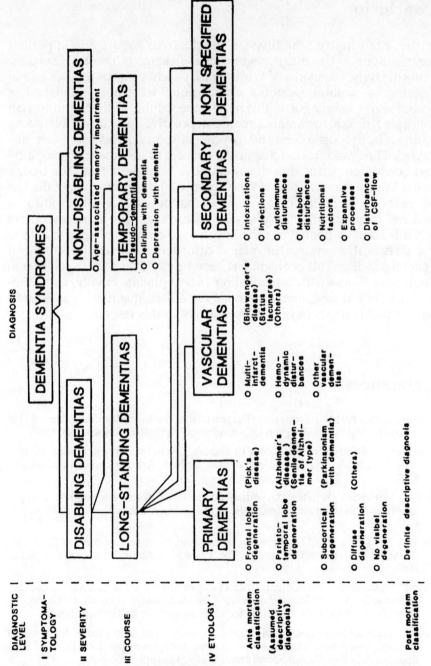

Figure 1. Diagram suggested by Gottfries (1988) for classification of dementia syndromes.

Conclusion

In the 20th century Scandinavian psychiatrists have made important contributions to the diagnosis and classification of mental disorders. Unfortunately, the works of Wimmer on psychogenic psychoses and of Sjöbring on multidimensional classification were only published in Scandinavian languages. In this review the validity of the Scandinavian concepts of schizophrenia, manic-depressive psychosis including schizo-affective disorders and psychogenic psychoses has been discussed. The Scandinavian diagnostic concept of neuroses, psychopathy and borderline personality disorders have been described. The design of the Danish classification systems of mental disorders during the last 50 years is currently being used in nationwide census studies of patients in psychiatric hospitals or institutions. As more and more patients are now treated outside hospitals, the time has come to extend the classification system of mental disorders to cover the setting of general practice. This problem has been briefly discussed in relation to depressive illness with somatization and to phobia. Finally, the standardized clinical assessment methods have been mentioned, as Scandinavian psychiatrists have also been active in this respect.

References

American Psychiatric Association: *Diagnostic and Statistical Manual of Mental Disorders (DSM-III)*. Washington DC. American Psychiatric Association, 1980.

Arentsen K, Strömgren E: Patients in Danish psychiatric hospitals. Results of a census in 1957. *Acta Jutlandica, Medical Series 9*, Århus, Universitetsforlaget, 1959.

Åsberg M, Perris C, Schalling D, Sedvall G: The CPRS, the development and applications of a psychiatric rating scale. *Acta Psychiatrica Scandinavica* 1978 (suppl. 271): 1–69.

Bech P: DSM-III and ICD-9: *Developments and levels of communicative validity. Psychometric and international perspective*. Clinical Update, Kalamazoo, Upjohn, 1987.

Bech P: Methodological problems in assessing quality of life as outcome in psychopharmacology. A multi-axial approach. In: *Methodology and evaluation of psychotropic drugs*, Benkert O, Rickels K (eds.). Springer, Berlin 1989 (in press).

Bech P, Kastrup M, Rafaelsen OJ: Mini-compendium of rating scales for states of anxiety, depression, mania, schizophrenia with corresponding DSM-III syndromes. *Acta Psychiatrica Scandinavica* 1986; 73 (suppl. 326):1–37.

Bech P, Hjortsø S, Lund K, Vilmar T, Kastrup M: An integration of the DSM-III and ICD-8 by global severity assessments for measuring multi-dimensional outcomes in general hospital psychiatry. *Acta Psychiatrica Scandinavica* 1987; 75:297-306.

Bech P, Allerup P, Gram LF, Kragh-Sørensen P, Rafaelsen OJ, Reisby N, Vestergaard P and DUAG: The Diagnostic Melancholia Scale (DMS): Dimensions of endogenous and reactive depression with relationship to the Newcastle Scales. *Journal of Affective Disorders* 1988; 14:161-170.

Christiansen H, Smith JC, Magnussen G: Report on the results of treatment with insulin shock. *Acta Psychiatrica et Neurologica* 1942; 17:221-235.

Committee on Forms and Statistics: *Statistical quide, State of New York, Department of Mental Hygiene*. New York, Utica: State Hospitals Press, Eleventh Edition, 1934.

Danish Psychiatric Association: *Diagnostic System of Mental Disorders*. Copenhagen, Danish Psychiatric Association 1938.

Danish Psychiatric Association: Diagnostic System of Mental Disorders (Diagnoseliste med kommentarer). *Nordisk Psykiatrisk Medlemsblad* 1952; 6:277-295. (English version published by Stengel, 1959).

Eberhard G, Ottosson JO: Icke-regressiv schizofreni. *Nordisk Psykiatrisk Tidsskrift* 1988; 4: 275-280.

Essen-Möller E: Suggestions for further improvement of the international classification of mental disorders. *Psychological Medicine* 1971; 1:308-311.

Essen-Möller E, Wohlfahrt S: Suggestions for the amendment of the official Swedish classification of mental disorders. *Acta Psychiatrica et Neurologica* 1947 (Suppl. 47): 551-555.

Færgeman PM: *De psykogene psykoser belyst gennem katamnestiske undersøgelser*. Copenhagen, Munksgaard 1945.

Færgeman PM: *Psychogenic psychoses. A description and follow-up of psychoses following psychological stress*. London: Butterworths 1963.

Goldberg DP, Bridges K: Somatic presentations of psychiatric illness in primary care setting. *Journal of Psychosomatic Research* 1988; 32: 137-144.

Gottesman II, Shields J: *Schizophrenia and genetics: A twin study vantage point*. New York, Academic Press, 1972.

Gottfries CG: *The definition and the classification of dementias*. Läkartidningen 1988 (in press).

Hamilton M: Development of a rating scale for primary depressive illness. *British Journal of Sociological and Clinical Psychology* 1967; 6: 278-296.

Helgason T: Epidemiology of mental disorders in Iceland. *Acta Psychiatrica Scandinavica* 1964; 40 (suppl. 173): 11-258.

Hoch PH, Polatin P: Pseudoneurotic forms of schizophrenia. *Psychiatry* 1949; 23: 248-276.

Hoche A: Die Bedeutung der Symptomenkomplexe in der Psychiatrie. *Zeitschrift Neurologie und Psychiatrie* 1912; 12: 540-551.

International Statistical Institute: *The International Classification of Diseases (ICD-4)*. Health Organization of the League of Nations, 1929.

International Statistical Institute: *The International Classification of Diseases (ICD-5)*. Health Organization of the League of Nations, 1938.

Jacobsen, E: *Psychoneuroser*. Copenhagen: Munksgaard, 1965.

Juel-Nielsen N, Strömgren E: Five years later. A comparison between census studies of patients in psychiatric institutions in Denmark in 1957 and 1962. *Acta Jutlandica, Medical Series 13*, Århus, Universitetsforlaget, 1963.

Jørgensen B, Nørrelund N, Bech P, Jacobsen K: Smerter og depressive symptomer i almen praksis. *Ugeskrift for Læger* 1984; 146: 2868–2872.

Kierkegaard S: *Begrebet angest*. Copenhagen, CA Reitzel, 1844.

Lange C: Bemærkninger om Grønlands sygdomsforhold. *Bibliotek for Læger* 1864; 5: 15–64.

Lange C: *Periodische Depressionszustände und ihre Pathogenesis auf dem Boden der harnsauren Diathese*. Leipzig: Verlag von Leopold Voss 1896 (Danish version 1886).

Marstal HB, Borup Svendsen B: An analysis of the doubling of admissions to Danish psychiatric institutions between 1948 and 1966. *Acta Jutlandica, Medical Series 15*, Århus, Universitetsforlaget, 1968.

Mors O: Increasing incidence of borderline states in Denmark from 1970-1985. *Acta Psychiatrica Scandinavica* 1988; 77: 575–583.

Munk-Jørgensen P: Why has the incidence of schizophrenia in Danish psychiatric institutions decreased since 1970? *Acta Psychiatrica Scandinavica* 1987; 75: 62–68.

Nyman GE: The clinical picture of non-regressive schizophrenia. *Nordisk Psykiatrisk Tidsskrift* 1975; 29: 249–258.

Nyman AK: Non-regressive schizophrenia. Clinical course and outcome. *Acta Psychiatrica Scandinavica* 1978 (suppl. 272).

Odegård O: *Diagnostic and classification tradition in Norway*, 1988.

Ottosson JO, Perris C: Multidimensional classification of mental disorders. *Psychological Medicine* 1973; 3: 238–243.

Perris C: A study of cycloid psychoses. *Acta Psychiatrica Scandinavica* 1974 (Suppl 153).

Pichot P: Psychopathic behaviour: A historical overview. In Hare RD, Schalling D (eds.): *Psychopathic behaviour: Approaches to research*. Chichester: John Wiley & Sons 1978, pp. 55–70.

Pichot P: Evaluation methods of the therapeutic effects of anxiety disorders treatment. In Pepplinkhuizen L, Verhoeven WMA (eds.): *Biological psychiatry in Europe today*. Leiderdorf: Vigeversig De Medicus 1986, pp. 69–73.

Pontoppidan K: Om den grønlandske kajaksvimmelhed. *Bibliotek for Læger* 1900; 93: 59–65.

Randløv C, Parnas G: The concept of borderline conditions among Danish psychiatrists. *Nordisk Psykiatrisk Tidsskrift* 1988; 42: 39–44.

Schneider K: *Psychopathic personalities*. London: Cassel 1958.

Sjöbring H: Mental constitution and mental illness. *Svenska Läkare Sällskap* 1919; 45: 462–493. (Translated by Essen-Möller in: Hirsch SR, Shepherd M (eds.): *Themes and variations in European psychiatry*. Bristol: John Wright & Sons 1974, pp. 265–294.

Slater E: Book review of P.M. Færgeman (1963). *British Journal of Psychiatry* 1964; 110: 114–118.

Stengel E: Classification of mental disorders. *Bulletin World Health Organization* 1959; 21: 601–663.

Strömgren E: Beiträge zur psychiatrischen Erblehre. *Acta Psychiatrica et Neurologica* 1938 (Suppl. 19).

Strömgren E: Psychogenic psychoses. In Hirsch SR, Shepherd M (eds): *Themes and variations in European psychiatry*. Bristol: John Wright & Sons 1974, pp. 97–117.

Strömgren E: The development of the concept of reactive psychoses. *Psychopathology* 1986; 20: 62–67.

Stürup GK, Smith JC, Hahnemann V: Report on the results of convulsion therapy. *Acta Psychiatrica et Neurologica* 1942; 17: 237–261.

Svendsen, Borup B: Psychiatric morbidity among civilians in wartime. *Acta Jutlandica Medical Series 8*, Århus: Universitetsforlaget 1952.

Sørensen BF: Om lette endogene depressioners klinik og behandling. *Månedsskrift for Praktisk Lægegerning* 1960; 38: 115–135.

Vanggaard T: Om schizofrene grænsetilstande. *Nordisk Psykiatrisk Medlemsblad* 1955; 9: 1–16.

Vanggaard T: *Borderlands of sanity*. Copenhagen: Munksgaard, 1979.

Wimmer A: Psykogene sindssygdomsformer. In *Sct. Hans Mental Hospital 1816–1916, Jubilee Publication*. Copenhagen: Gad 1916 pp. 85–216.

Wing JK, Cooper JE, Sartorius N: *The measurement and classification of psychiatric symptoms*. Cambridge: Cambridge University Press, 1974.

World Health Organization: *Manual of the International Statistical Classification of Diseases, Injuries, and Causes of Death (ICD-6)*. Bulletin World Health Organization, 1948 (Suppl. 1).

World Health Organization: *Manual of the International Classification of Diseases (ICD-7)*. Geneva: World Health Organization, 1955.

World Health Organization: *Manual of the International Classification of Diseases (ICD-8)*. Geneva: World Health Organization, 1967.

World Health Organization: *Report of the international pilot study of schizophrenia*. Geneva: World Health Organization, 1973.

World Health Organization: *Report on the WHO collaborative study on standardized assessment of depressive disorders*. Geneva: World Health Organization, 1983.

World Health Organization: *Glossary of mental disorders and guide to their classification for use in conjunction with the International Classification of Diseases. Eighth Revision*. Geneva: World Health Organization, 1974.

World Health Organization: Mental disorders: *Glossary and guide to their classification in accordance with the Ninth Revision of the International Classification of Diseases*. Geneva: World Health Organization, 1978.

7
On the Forms of Development in Mental Disorders

A. V. Snezhnevsky†*

As stated by Zeller (1840), the development of nosological concepts in psychiatry depends on the success of studying the course of disturbances. "The succession of the changing symptoms corresponds to the course of pathological processes," and further, "the clinical task is to distinguish the succession of symptoms which is typical for the given psychopathological process" [1]. Several decades later the same idea was developed by Kahlbaum: "A natural development of a disease lies in the variety of its course, embracing the illness from the beginning till the end of its development" [2]. Later still, in 1906, V.P. Serbsky substantiated this statement as follows: "It is necessary to distinguish states representing just one of the periods in the development of a morbid process from the illness itself which is comprised of several states representing a known and often quite certain and consecutive course of development. Only the study of the development mode from its beginning to the end, only the whole complex of the clinical course of the process can provide a complete picture of the illness itself" [3]. The same was mentioned by E. Kraepelin in the latest period of his work [4]. He pointed out in particular that the forms of dementia praecox course described by him represent not the forms of disease themselves (nicht von eigentlichen Formen) but pictures of states (Zustandsbildern), usually protracted. It can be added that K. Jaspers [5] has also substantiated the necessity of carefully recorded patients' histories containing descriptions of the disturbance development from its onset up to the end.

However, the possibility of investigating all peculiarities of the disease manifestations throughout its full development remains, in the great majority of cases in most countries, unfeasible. This can be achieved only if, besides hospitals and clinics, there is a well-developed system of outpatient psychiatric care which maintains non-stop medical psychiatric monitoring of the patients' full illness from its onset

---

* Institute of Psychiatry of the Academy of Medical Sciences of the USSR, Moscow, USSR.

throughout the treatment course and up until the rehabilitation period. In other words, it is possible to investigate mental illnesses only if besides mental hospitals there exists an outpatient psychiatric assistance system providing for continuous supervision and treatment of mental patients at home. Provided there exists a long-term outpatient psychiatric institution in a given region, a nearly complete screening of all mentally disturbed individuals living there is achieved.

To investigate the illness in its development is the only way to overcome static syndromology, which excludes the possibility of studying the dynamics of the process and thus disclosing its intrinsic regularities, interfering with its dynamics and forecasting the outcome. P.B. Gannushkin in his time complained that in psychiatry too much attention was paid to the study and analysis of the patient's "state" and so little was said about the "course" of the illness [6]. Meanwhile, the specificity of the illness is expressed through its successive development, i.e., through its pathokinetic specificity [7].

Investigating any illness in its development makes it possible to discover the presence of its three inherent qualities: "specific," "separate," and "unitary."

The "specific" of all mental disorders represents a stable quality distinguishing this disorder. This is displayed particularly by the form of its course—continuously progressive, attack-like progressive, periodical, stepwise (phasic). In this connection, the form of an illness is mentioned, which essentially is the form of the course of a disorder. The form preserves its generic qualities from the onset up to the end of the illness [8]. The constancy in form of the disease course is provided by the so-called major pathogenetic disorder. Clinical manifestations of the illness through their "own language" and own laws of development inform about the motive forces in the pathological process. Progression is displayed through the clinical picture getting more complicated. Primarily the complex constellation of the "inner conditions" of the disorder determines an extraordinary variability of forms in mental illnesses.

Unlike the "specific," the "separate" quality of a disorder is changeable.

If determining the variety of an illness, for instance, schizophrenia proceeded by attacks from onset till the end ("specific" quality) can have various manifestations. Its first attack can be in the form of oneiroid catatonia, whereas the ones to follow are limited to depressive or manic disorders. In other cases the initial attack can be depressive-paranoid, the next—in a disorder in the form of Mandinsky-Clerambaut syndrome and the ones to develop later—with prevailing catatonic symptoms. Together with the modes already mentioned, cases are not infrequently found with attacks of the same mode—manic only, or in the form of acute paranoia, etc.

The distinctions of attack-like course of an illness shown here allow one to point out three varieties of the "separate" feature of illness—regressive, progressive, stationary.

Together with the qualities of an illness already considered, in every case of any illness one discovers its "singular," i.e., individual, manifestations. They originate within the framework of the "specific" and the "separate," but with qualities inherent only in this given patient. This relates not only to the contents of pathological phenomena, but also to their form. We can speak of individual manifestations of hallucinations, delusions, syndrome of influence, etc.

Investigation of an illness in view of the three above-mentioned aspects (specific, separate and singular) is reflected through descriptive diagnosis—illness, its form, variety, and individual features. Thus, major peculiarities of an illness, its general and individual qualities are contained in a descriptive diagnosis. It is distinguished from the so-called multiaxial diagnosis, which contains multiple, various but equalized signs of pathology.

By studying the illness in its development from the onset to end it is possible to overcome rigid syndromology, to investigate the dynamics of the morbid process and to disclose its intrinsic laws; also the ways opening up for intervention and prognostication of the outcome are revealed. In other words, the study of all peculiarities in the course of an illness underlies the existing classification of disorders and their separate forms.

In the study of the course of schizophrenia conducted in one of Moscow's districts using epidemiological methods, the following data were found:

Table 1. Schizophrenic illness distribution in the population (per 1000 people)'[9].

Form	Incidence	Prevalence	%
Malignant	0.008	0.54	6.0
Progressive	0.027	1.95	11.6
Slowly progressive	0.082	3.47	38.4
Attack-like progressive	0.042	2.77	30.6
Recurrent	0.030	2.20	13.4
Total	0.19	10.93	100.0

From the data shown in the table it follows primarily that forms of the course of schizophrenia do not correspond to observed Kraepelin "state pictures." According to these data, sluggish and attack-like progressive forms of schizophrenia are the most common ones (69%).

Varieties of schizophrenia with an unfavorable course (malignant and progressive) constitute 17.60% of all cases of schizophrenia.

Continuous and attack-like forms of the course of schizophrenia constitute 56% and 44%, respectively. However, this distribution is relative. In a proposition of cases the above-mentioned forms initially develop as one-two attacks, whereas further development of the disease becomes seemingly continuous, albeit with expressed exacerbations being present. Shubform development of the process can change over to forms with a phasic course. In continuously proceeding forms there may be a tendency for an attack-like course.

A change of shubs (i.e., shifts) which proceed on the background of an increasing defect after every attack by phases (exacerbations of illness with a prevailing affective disorder without an increase of the defect) is apparently suggestive of an emerging compensation and of a stabilization at the level of an existing mental defect. Such compensation is usually unstable and may be interrupted by destabilization flashes.

Unlike other forms, in malignant continuous schizophrenia such relative stabilization does not develop until the final state.

The above-mentioned regularities in the development of the process determine individual peculiarities of the illness. Individual differences in malignant forms are not great. They are discovered only in the duration of catatonic-type exacerbations, in some qualities of verbal pseudo-hallucinations during remissions in disease manifestations, in the peculiarities of fragmentary delusions, behavioral mannerisms (prosectic, negativistic) and other phenomena. In the progressive variety of schizophrenia with an unfavorable course, many more varieties are found. In some cases various manifestations of Kandinsky-Clerambaut syndrome prevail, in others varieties of paraphrenic delusions. In both cases there is a prevalence of either delusional disorders or pseudohallucinations. Exacerbations are accompanied either by an intensification of the mentioned disorders or by emerging catatonic agitation.

Slowly progressive (torpid) form of schizophrenia is more frequently monomorphous in its manifestation, its course may be in the form of persistent obsessions, cenestopathic disorders, hypochondriasis, asthenic, hysterical or paranoiacal disorders. It is accompanied by slowly developing symptoms of a schizophrenic defect in the form of autism, emotional impoverishment, sometimes by regressive symptoms, all the time with phenomena of an energetic potential drop. This variety includes the so-called simple form. Some authors attribute varieties of slowly progressive forms of schizophrenia to the so-called intermediate form, the course of which sometimes resembles a psychosis and sometimes neurosis.

In its clinical characteristics, the range of attack-like progressive schizophrenia manifestations is the most diversified. It ranges from various types of acute catatonic (paranoid, depressive, confused, oneiroid), to depressive-paranoid, depressive-hallucinatory, acute paraphrenia, acute hallucinosis and pseudohallucinosis, and acute paranoia. All the disorders enumerated are as a rule imaginative, sensuous, total and polymorphous. Delusions in this form are sensuous, where not only rationality, but also sensual cognition is disturbed. Here one doesn't find any consistent system of proofs. Its contents are dominated by imaginative conceptions and plastic sensuality (imaginations, fantasies, dreams). Delusional conceptions in these cases are extremely fragmentary, containing much uncertainty and inconsistency. The contents of imaginative delusions can be closer to real events or absolutely fantastic. It is accompanied by perplexity. Infrequently, suddenness and inconsistency is predominate in the patient's actions. The personality changes usually appear after the first attack. In cases with a tendency toward progression, the defect can increase to the degree of a marked drop in energetic potential, sometimes with residual symptoms during remission. In most cases after the first acute attack, the change becomes stable, and further attacks of illness proceed not in the form of shubs (shifts) but in phases. In a number of cases, the cause of the illness becomes not progressive but regressive. In such cases, after the first or second attack, which proceed with marked catatonic, catatonic-oneiroid or depressive-paranoid disorders, further attacks develop as affective depressive or manic, more frequently circular.

In attack-like progressive and also in recurrent forms of schizophrenia there are not infrequent cases with a singular attack course, where one attack is followed by a lengthy (over 25 years) remission and only slight personality changes. According to our data, in patients with attack-like progressive and recurrent schizophrenia lasting over 15 years, the frequency of a singular attack course is as follows: with course duration from 15 to 24 years—32.8%, from 25 to 40 years—30%, over 40 years duration—23.9%.

K. Conrad [10] and a number of other authors have also divided the course of cadogenous psychoses into four types: continuously progressive, progressive in the form of attacks, remittent and cyclothymic. The most favorably proceeding attack-like progressive and also recurrent-form schizophrenias are related by some researchers not to its processual variety but to schizophrenic reactions (episodes). However, there is a reservation that some transitory disorders turn into psychotic processes [11]. The course of recurrent forms of schizophrenia is on the verge of intermittent. Attacks of a recurrent form are intensive in their manifestations, always being accompanied by a marked effect. Their clinical picture is diverse: intensive oneiroid disorders, fantastic-paraphrenic or circular (depressions or manic states with sensuous delusions, singular illusions or hallucinations). Some authors relate the recurrent form, especially its circular varieties, to cyclothymia. Inherent in the latent forms of schizophrenia is the change of personal traits distinctive of this illness (autism, emotional poverty, decrease of capacity for work to a certain degree or, on the contrary, machine-like activity). Under the influence of one or another factors, quick transitory psychotic episodes are possible. Over the years personality traits may be intensified, though this does not happen in all cases. Because of difficulties in diagnosing and also in view of many cases escaping the attention of specialists, the nature of such forms remains unclear. Residual schizophrenia as a rule is hardly distinguishable from latent schizophrenia as well as from protracted remission. The differentiation of residual disorders from manifestations of permission is far from perfect. In theory, latent and residual schizophrenia could be related to the pathos and not to the nozos category [12], that is, if by pathos we understand the presence of pathogenetic mechanisms of an illness, a kind of diathesis, readiness for the development of pronounced forms of an illness; and by nozos the morbid process itself in all its clinical expression.

As substantiated by modern investigations, the course of cyclothymia (manic-depressive psychosis) is no less diverse than that of schizophrenia. As we know, there can be only depressive or only manic phases (monopolar course) as well as circular disorders with changing manic and depressive phases (bipolar course). Among psychoses, manic-depressive psychosis is found much less than schizophrenia. Table 2 shows corresponding data for 3 districts of Moscow [13].

Table 2. Distribution of patients with endogenous psychoses.

Illness	Abs.	%
Schizophrenia	5073	94.8
Manic-depressive psychosis	278	5.2
Total	5351	100.0

Specific features of the development of manic-depressive psychosis are shown in Table 3.

Genetic studies have also demonstrated a closeness between recurrent schizophrenia and manic-depressive psychosis.

The incidence of periodical endogenous psychoses in the population (recurrent schizophrenia and manic-depressive psychosis) is 1.59 per 1000 population, where figures for recurrent schizophrenia incidence

Table 3. Distribution of patients with manic-depressive psychosis according to type of illness course.

Course type	Number of patients	
	Absol.	%
Circular (bipolar)	52	19.0
Periodical depressions	179	65.3
Periodical manias	0	0
Singular depressions	43	15.7
Singular manias	0	0
TOTAL	274	100.0

are 2.5 times higher than those for manic-depressive psychosis—1.13 and 0.45 per 1000 population, respectively. Monopolar (more frequently, depressive) forms of manic-depressive psychosis are found consistently more often than bipolar ones (0.33 and 0.12 per 1000 population, respectively). Manic-depressive psychosis takes its course in the population mainly in an outpatient environment, for incidence, of psychotic forms only 0.13 per 1000. Conversely, schizo-affective psychoses are mainly characterized by the manifested psychotic course, and their outpatient varieties are exceptionally rare (0.07 per 1000).

In manic-depressive psychosis and recurrent schizophrenia, depressive states are the most widely spread, comprising 82% of all affective phases in manic-depressive psychosis and over 50% of all psychotic states in patients with recurrent schizophrenia.

In the female population manic-depressive psychosis affection is four times higher, and schizo-affective psychosis affection twice as high as in the male population. The highest morbidity levels in population were observed in the age group 60–69 years and for the recurrent form from 40–49 years of age.

In 70% of the patients with manic-depressive psychosis, affective psychoses are manifested after 40 years of age, and in 98.2% of cases, the clinical picture is that of depressive syndromes. Manic debuts of manic-depressive psychosis are extremely rare, but with every successive attack the proportion of manic states increases.

The above-mentioned regularities of the illness course which are expressed through their clinical forms naturally inhere not only in endogenous psychoses, but also in all mental illnesses. But together with form diversity of psychosis there is also the common character of their manifestations. In the course of many nosologically different psychoses similar varieties of clinical disorders can emerge, marked by positive ("plus") symptoms (e.g., in circular, agitated, polymorphous forms) and of by negative ("minus") symptoms (simple forms of various mental illnesses) [14]; the latter represent the most specific nosological manifestation of mental illness.

Diversity in forms of the course is inherent in all mental illness. It is determined primarily by the intrinsic qualities of the disease-stricken organism. In this connection reference can be made to the words of the renowned Soviet pathologist I.V. Davidovsky, who maintained that "external factors can engender in an organism or provoke in it nothing that it already doesn't have as historically developed potencies. Whatever external factors might be, they can evoke only appropriate, i.e., adequate to them, changes in the organism, which means that in the organism itself there should be 'intrinsic base' for such changes" [15].

Such a view can be supported by observed peculiarities in the course of familial schizophrenias. As a rule, there is similarity, i.e., certain constancy, of the illness course in a proband and his or her relatives. The similarity of forms of mental illness course in the family favors its endogenous conditionality. At the same time, apparently, absolute subdivision of mental pathology into endogenous and exogenous processes is somewhat artificial. Not without reason did Maudsley say in his time: "Nature does not recognize those artificial and ill-fated subdivisions which are created for convenience and not infrequently in the interests of ignorance." One can be sure that as our knowledge of the nature of mental disorder develops, we shall be able to have more exact notions regarding the interrelationships of internal and external disease factors as well as of the role of functional readiness which determines predispositions, i.e., the possibility for one or another pathological processes to develop.

References

1) Cit. Ju. V. Kannabikh, *Istoriya psikhiatrii*, 1928, p. 263

2) Ibid. p. 408

3) V.P. Serbsky, *Zhurnal nevropatologii i piskhiatrii im.* Korsakova, 1906, No. 3.

4) Cit. L. Voigt, Über Dementia praecox in Kindesalter. *Zeitsch. J. Neurol. u. Psych.* 3d. 8, 1919, p. 225.

5) K. Jaspers, *Allgemeine Psychopathologie.* 6. Auflage, 1953, 5, 506–516.

6) P. B. Gannushkin. *Selected works*, Moscow, 1964.

7) I.V. Davidovsky, *Problemy prichinnosti v meditsine*, Moscow, 1962.

8) Ibid.

9) Tabulated data on the forms of disease courses shown here and below have been introduced by Dr. L.M. Schmaonova, Head of the Epidemiology Department at the Institute of Psychiatry.

10) K. Conrad. Das Problem der "Nosologischen Einheit" in der Psychiatrie. *Der Nervenarzt*, 1959, II, 1488.

11) H. Krüger. *Die Schizophrenie*. P. Enke Verlag. Stuttgart, 1981.

12) I. Vertkin. "Nozologia," *Bolshaya Meditsinskaya Encyclopaedia*, p. 88–89, 1961.

13) The figures shown in Table 3 also relate to three districts of Moscow.

14) The presence of pathologically positive and negative features in manifestations of each mental disorder was originally mentioned by Monroe in 1851.

15) I.V. Davidovsky, *Problemy prichinnosti v meditsine*, Moscow, 1962.

8

The Third-World Perspective on Psychiatric Diagnosis and Classification

N. N. Wig*

There is no standard definition of the term "Third World," but it is generally accepted that it refers to the majority of the countries in Asia, Africa and Latin America, distinguishing them from industrially developed countries. In the field of health and social development, most of the countries of the Third World have many common features including low per capita income, low life expectancy, high population growth and a poorly established system of modern health services.

The Third World has been the home of some of the world's oldest cultures with traditions going back for thousands of years. It also contains nearly three quarters of the world's mentally ill. It would be presumptuous to speak on behalf of the entire Third World with its many countries, cultures and subcultures. Thus, it must be stated at the outset that the present author's background and familiarity is mostly with South East Asia and the Eastern Mediterranean Region. This bias is bound to be reflected in subsequent discussion.

Sources and Traditions of Medicine in the Third World

In the Third World, there are at present at least three major medical traditions, those of (1) China and the Far East, (2) India and South Asia, and (3) the Islamic and Arab countries of the Middle East and North Africa. In Latin American countries, time has brought about a mixture of European traditions and remnants of many earlier indigenous civilizations, e.g., those of the Mayas, the Incas and the Aztecs. Sub-Saharan Africa has its own rich cultures and traditions, less uniformly spread in the many countries that compose it.

---

* Regional Adviser Mental Health, World Health Organization, Eastern Mediterranean Regional Office, Alexandria, Egypt.

The Chinese and Indian civilizations have a continuous history of more than 3000 years. Islamic history is also now nearly 1400 years old. Each one of these major civilizations, particularly Chinese, Indian and Islamic, have a rich heritage and traditions in various branches of sciences and arts like mathematics, astronomy, architecture, music and literature. They have also a very long and continuous historical tradition in medicine with hundreds of medical texts preserved from the past. There are hundreds of thousands of practitioners of medicine which was traditional in these civilizations. In India alone, it was estimated that in 1966 there were more than 400,000 practitioners of the traditional systems of medicines, as compared with only 86,000 practitioners of modern medicine (Rao, 1966).

In addition to the practitioners of traditional medical systems in these countries, there are numerous religious healers or faith healers also providing help to people for psychological and psychosocial problems. They are a large and heterogeneous group. Some of them use magical and occult practices. They may make astrological predictions, use trance-like experience in which spirits are supposed to "possess" the healers or the sufferer, and use various means to remove the evil spirits or the effects of a curse. Others in this group are members of the priestly class or leaders of the established religious order, to whom people go for advice and counseling, and who on the basis of prevailing religious teachings provide psychological counseling. There is considerable overlap between practices used by the various groups. Some religious leaders use amulets and other magical symbols. Removal of evil spirits has been practiced in the shrines associated with almost all major religions. Religious healers also use herbal medicines. Common to all the religious and faith healers, however, are a belief system shared by the healer and the patient and the culturally approved, powerful personality of the healer.

In the countries of the Third World, the spiritual and religious varieties of healing still play a very significant part in the management of psychiatric and psychosocial disorders. Native healers using magic and occult practices are widespread in the countries of Africa and parts of Asia. In many Islamic countries (e.g., Sudan) religious healers are very prominent members of the society, particularly in rural areas (Baasher, 1975). In India and Pakistan, thousands of mentally ill and their relatives visit shrines, usually established on the graves of saints and holy men.

There is no doubt that beliefs about magic and witchcraft, traditional and religious healing exist in the industrially developed countries as well; a senior French psychiatrist has estimated that in France there are more practitioners of traditional medicine (e.g., herbalists, magnetizers, etc.) than there are practitioners who have received training in an approved school of modern medicine. However, these practices are somehow not in the social mainstream and are kept somewhat secret. In contrast, in the Third World, religious and traditional medicine and its practitioners are widely accepted. The majority of the people with psychotic disorders who reach mental health services have visited more than one traditional healer before they come to the psychiatrist. Similarly, symptoms of spirit possession are not uncommon in the psychiatric clinics of developing countries, and such symptoms are regularly seen against the background of a manic, schizophrenic or hysterical disorder.

Although most countries of the world accept modern scientific medicine as the basis for their public health action as well as for their preventive and curative medical services, in many countries of the Third World the governments also provide patronage and financial support to other well-established traditional systems. These include the Chinese traditional medicine (including acupuncture) in China, Ayurveda in India, Sri Lanka and countries of South Asia, and Unani or Arabic medicine in India, Pakistan and other countries in the Middle East. Some African countries recognize and support traditional healers' associations. In many of these countries there are government-funded colleges and hospitals based on these systems and separate sections in the ministries of health entrusted with their development. Governments support research on methods of traditional medicine and on possibilities of its linkage with the modern scientific medical system. Nongovernmental organizations and private institutions are also found among those supporting traditional medicine in these countries.

Finally, there are numerous other systems of medicine in both developed and developing countries which claim a "scientific" basis and have a degree of popular acceptance. Some of them, like homeopathy and osteopathy, have won official recognition, and some countries have established standards of qualifications for the practice of such forms of medicine and support colleges providing training in their application.

It must be emphasized that no one medical system—whether it is called scientific or pseudo-scientific—has ever fulfilled the needs and aspirations of all human beings. There have always been parallel systems of medicines based on a variety of theories with a differing amount of evidence supporting them. The existence of various types of psychotherapies and clinics promising enhancement of health and quality of life are among the more recent examples of this phenomenon.

Existing Organized Traditional Systems of Medicine in the Third World

Under the influence of European colonial powers, modern scientific medicine spread to the countries of Asia and Africa only relatively recently. Slowly, the benefits of modern scientific medicine started becoming obvious, and almost every country in the world has by now adopted this as the official basis for its practice of health care, especially in the promotion of public health. However, this has not meant an elimination of the older traditional systems, which continue to enjoy great popularity among the people in many countries. In the majority of countries of the Third World, modern medical hospitals and clinics are available only for a small proportion of the urban populations. For the vast rural sections of the population, as well as for the poorer urban sections, the health service facilities are either nonexistent or inadequate, so that the people have to look toward practitioners of traditional systems of medicine for help.

After the Second World War, almost all countries of Asia and Africa attained independence from colonial rule. This has brought about a new awareness of the existing traditional systems in the field of health and social development. In these developing countries, on the one hand, there is a desire for quick modernization of the traditional societies and for rapidly reaping the benefits of modern scientific knowledge and technology. On the other hand, with the attainment of political independence, there is usually a great upsurge of national and regional pride in the existing cultures. There has been a great revival of cultural heritage of the past in art, music, literature and sciences, particularly in those countries in which civilizations have been continuous—e.g., in China, India or the Islamic countries. In these countries, a common intellectual preoccupation is to seek answers to the question of how to bring in modern scientific technology without simultaneously introducing the value system of Western Europe and North America.

Traditional Medical Systems in India and South East Asia

In India and the neighboring countries, like Nepal, Bangladesh and Sri Lanka, a highly developed and elaborate system of medicine has flourished for nearly three thousand years. It is generally known by the name of *Ayurveda* (the sciences of life). The Arabic system of medicine was also introduced in India during the time of Muslim empires and enjoyed court patronage under the Muslim rulers. It soon became popular among the general population. In India, it is known by the name of *Tib-E-Unani* or *Unani* (Greek) medicine (see below).

After the independence of India, Sri Lanka, Pakistan, Bangladesh and other countries in South-East Asia, there was a great resurgence of interest in Ayurveda and Unani medicine, though all the countries of this region have accepted the modern scientific medicine and modern public health system for the government health services. In India, Bangladesh, Sri Lanka, etc, there are now government-funded dispensaries, hospitals, colleges and research institutions based on these traditional systems. There are provisions for separate registration of these practitioners. In India, there are separate medical councils for Ayurveda and Unani medicine.

Psychological Concepts in Ayurveda

There are many medical texts dating back to the 1st or 2nd century A.D. which describe in detail the principles of Ayurveda. Over the centuries, numerous commentaries have been written by successive generations of Ayurvedic physicians (Jolly, 1977). The two best known medical works are by the Ayurvedic physicians Caraka and Susruta. These are probably the most often quoted Indian medical texts. These books were originally compiled sometime between the 3rd century B.C. to the 3rd century A.D. *Caraka Simhata* is generally regarded as the older of the two. *Susruta Simhata* also has a section on surgical diseases which is missing in Caraka's book.

The principles of Ayurvedic medicine, like in other Indian philosophical systems, were probably well developed by the 6th century B.C. There is a close similarity between the ancient Indian and Greek thought, particularly in the fields of astronomy, mathematics, religion and medicine, though there were no clear historical contacts between two civilizations till the invasion of India by Alexander the Great in 326 B.C. In Ayurveda the fundamental principle of health is the proper balance between five elements (*Bhutas*) and three humours (*Dosas*). The balance occurs at different levels: physical, physiological, psychological and finally spiritual—the state of bliss in which the ultimate goal is tranquility (Mora, 1980). The human being is considered an integral part of the nature and is made of the same five elements that constitute the universe, namely, water, air, fire, earth and sky. The three humours or Dosas recognized in Ayurvedic medicine are *Kaph* (phlegm), *Pitta* (bile) and *Vata* (wind). These terms for the three Dosas are still popularly used by people in India to describe the states of health and disease. In addition to the harmony and balance of three Dosas, it is recognized that for a healthy state, digestion should be normal, excretion of waste products should be unimpaired, and the person should be endowed with tranquility and clarity of senses, mind and soul. There are also clear references to indicate that the mind (*Manas*) can impair the state of health even if the senses (*Indriyas*), humours (*Dosas*) and elements (*Bhutas*) are functioning normally (Narayana-Reddy et al., 1987). However, the concept of *Manas* is not equal to the concept of mind in modern psychology and current usage. *Manas*, according to Caraka, is *Ate-indriya* or a kind of suprasensory organ that coordinates the input from senses (*Indriyas*) (Balodhi, 1987). There is another important mental concept, *Buddhi* (discriminating intellect or the faculty of judgment), which is generally considered to be higher than *Manas*. It must, however, be appreciated that the body/mind dichotomy that is so central to modern psychiatry is not essential to Ayurvedic thought. On the other hand, the separation between body and soul (*Atma*) is of much greater importance.

Another concept that is very central to Ayurvedic medicine and Indian philosophy is the *Tri-guna* or the theory of three inherent qualities or modes of nature. These three are *Sattva* (variously translated as light, goodness or purity), *Rajas* (action, energy, passion) and *Tamas* (darkness, inertia). In the medical and religious texts, the theory of three *gunas* is used repeatedly to describe different types of personalities, food, action, etc. For example, according to the Bhagawad Gita, the best known of Hindu religious books, a "Sattvic" person, who desires true knowledge and purity, is detached from his or her actions and is balanced. The "Rajasik" person is full of activity, passion and restlessness, while a "Tamsik" person is dull, lazy and indifferent.

Psychiatric Diagnosis and Classification in Ayurveda

All the major Ayurvedic texts like Carak Samhita and Susruta Simhata have a separate section dealing with insanity (*Unmada*). In addition, there are chapters on spirit possession (*bhutonmada*) and epilepsy (*apasmara*). Different types of convulsions, paralysis, fainting, intoxications are also well described. There is detailed description of different types of spirit possessions. Twenty-one sub-types based on three groups of *sattava, rajas,* and *tamas* are described. Though at times the descriptions appear artificial, some of them have clear resemblance to some modern descriptions of personality disorders, psychosis, and mental retardation (Dube, 1978).

The chapters on *unmada* (insanity) are very well written, both in Carak Samhita and Susruta Samhita. Six types of mental disorder are well recognized:

— *vatonmad* caused by *vata* dosa

— *kaphonmad* caused by *kapha* dosa

— *pittonmad* caused by *pitta* dosa

— *sampottonmad* caused by combined dosas

— *vishaja unmad* caused by external intoxications and poisons

— *shokaja unmad* caused by excessive grief.

In recent years, many psychiatrists in India have made serious attempts to equate some of these Ayurvedic descriptions to modern psychiatric diagnostic terms (Deb Sikdar, 1961; Varma, 1965; Dube, 1978). Unfortunately, the results are neither uniform nor comparable. What has been called a typical picture of schizophrenia by one author is considered as representative of manic-depressive psychosis or organic psychosis by the other authors. Weiss (1977) has summed up the position very well in the following lines:

> The relationship between specific Ayurvedic categories and present day nosological terms is often complex. The assumption of one-to-one correspondence between nosologies of two systems is overly simplistic. On the other hand, there do seem to be some elements of human condition, its pathology and psychopathology that are cross-culturally invariant. While recognizing that these comparisons fall short of an equation, one can nevertheless identify distinct examples or recognizable clinical entities in Ayurvedic literature.

In Ayurveda there are no separate chapters on neurosis or stress-related somatic illness. (Even in European psychiatry these concepts are relatively new, and most terms now used were introduced in the 20th century.) However, in Ayurveda there are numerous references that suggest that the influence of the psychological and environmental factors on health and disease was well recognized (Narayana-Reddy et al., 1987). Some modern writers (e.g., Ramu et al., 1988) have tried to identify separate neurotic conditions in Ayurveda like *atatwa bhinevesha* as obsession or *apatanaka* or *apatantraka* as hysteria or *chittodvega* as anxiety, but these are mostly used as descriptive terms and cannot be accepted as disease entity in a modern psychiatric sense. It must be remembered that Sanskrit—the language of Ayurveda—is a highly complex language in which the same word can have many shades of meanings.

The academic interest in Ayurveda is steadily increasing. There are many colleges and university departments in India and Sri Lanka and Nepal in which translations of old texts have been produced and commentaries written in the light of modern scientific knowledge. The National Institute of Mental Health and Neurosciences (NIMHANS) in Bangalore, India, has, since its inception in 1955, a separate Ayurvedic Research Unit. In recent years, a number of very good papers in English on various aspects of mental health in Ayurveda and Indian philosophy have been published in *NIMHANS Journal*.

Arabic or Islamic Medicine

Health sciences greatly flourished during the rise of Islamic civilization between the 7th and 12th centuries in the Middle East, Central Asia, North Africa and Spain. The Arab or Islamic medical system is still widely practiced in Pakistan, India and many Arab countries of the Middle East and Africa, particularly in the rural areas. It is difficult to choose an appropriate name for this medical system. Both terms, "Arabic" and "Islamic Medicine," alone do not seem fully justified because many pioneers of this system of medicine were not Arabs and sometimes not even Muslim. However, an "Arab" according to the Islamic tradition is a man whose language is Arabic—and all of these pioneers wrote in Arabic, which was used widely while this system of medicine was at its peak. In the Indian subcontinent, this system of medicine is called *Tib-E-Unani* or "Greek Medicine," which suggests its early roots yet again seem inappropriate in the present context. Khayat (1981) suggested the compromise term "Arab-Islamic Medicine."

Islamic Medicine has borrowed heavily from many sources. The original source was the existing Greek medical knowledge based on the theories of Hippocrates and Galen and other well-known scholars. The Greek medical texts reached the Islamic empire in Baghdad through Egypt and Syria. Islamic medicine has also been influenced greatly by Indian medical texts. During the early Islamic centuries, numerous medical texts from Greece and India were translated into Arabic. Soon the famous physicians belonging to the Arabic tradition, like Al Razi (Rhazes, 865–925 A.D.) and Ibn Sena (Avicena, 980–1037 A.D.), not only refined the old medical knowledge, but also gave it the present shape. The Arabic medical books, particularly Avicena's *Canon of Medicine*, had a deep impact on European medical traditions. It was an essential medical text in many universities in Europe until the 17th century.

Psychiatric Aspects of an Islamic Medicine

In the Islamic tradition the social attitude toward the mentally ill is based on the saying of Prophet Muhamad, that the mentally ill are dear to God. Some of the earliest hospitals in the world for the mentally ill were started in Baghdad and other Islamic cities where the patients were humanely treated (Baasher, 1975). In Cairo, in the 14th century, the Kalawoun hospital is known to have had four sections, one each for medical patients, surgical patients, eye patients and mental patients. This was perhaps the first example of a general hospital psychiatric unit (Baasher, 1975; Okasha, 1988).

In Arabic medicine, the concept of mind and mental illness is roughly comparable to the writing in earlier Greek classics. The soul is regarded as an entity separate from the body, and many psychological and moral attributes are linked with the soul. Al Razi, who first wrote his famous encyclopedic medical text, *Al Hawi*, on the various aspects of diseases and their cures, later wrote a comparable text on the ills of the soul and their treatment called *Tib-E-Ruhani* (Medicine of the Soul).

In Arab medical texts, the classification of psychiatric disorders generally follow the pattern in earlier Greek texts. Conditions like epilepsy, dementia, melancholia and hysteria are described. It is interesting to note that though the famous physician Constatinus Africanus (1020–1087) of the Salerno School (near Naples, Italy) is generally attributed to have separated two types of melancholias—one having its site in the brain and the other in the hypochondrium (Mora, 1980)—there is also a similar description in the writings of the Arabic physician Haly Abbas, who lived before Africanus, in the second half of the 10th century. Haly Abbas, in his book *Kamil-us-Sinaa* classified mental disorders in the following way:

1.   MELANCHOLY
1.1   due to an affection in the brain
1.2   due to an affection in other organs, with a brain involvement
a.   hypochondria
b.   due to vapors from burning humours (blood, phlegm, bile, black bile)
1.3   Melancholic obsession

2.   QUTRUB
Probably a type of insanity resembling present day schizophrenia. The description is that of grossly disturbed behaviour, with irrelevant talk and tendency to wander near graveyards, etc.

3.   ISHQ
Mental illness caused by unfulfilled romantic love. The description is usually of love-lorn youth, dejected in love.

The later well-known Arabic medical writers like Samarqandi (died 1227) have also used similar systems of classification. Some have included the conditions like delirium, epilepsy, paralysis, and vertigo in the chapter on mental disorders.

In the medical works of Ibn Jazlah written in the 11th century, there is a beautiful example of Arabic art of medical description and calligraphy (Graziani, 1980). The section on mental disorders consists of a one-page table that concisely describes the names of eight common mental disorders (melancholy, qutrub, ishq, etc.) on one side, while on the other side there are listed the aspects of disease like age, sex, season, causes, symptoms, management, etc. In the limited space of one page, almost all the relevant known facts have been summarized (see the following Arabic table and the English translation).

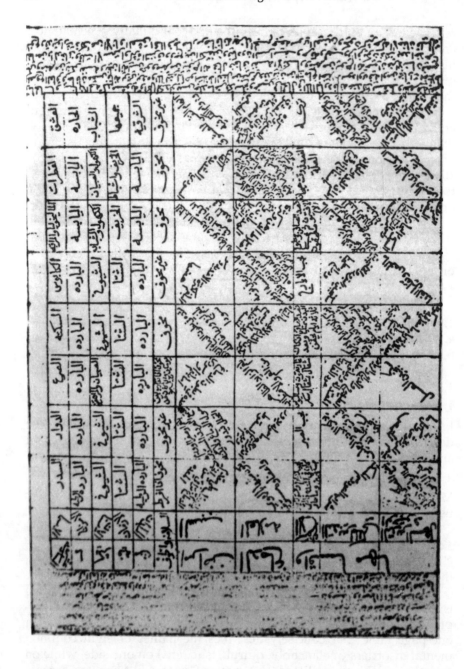

A table of mental illnesses, their description and their treatment from the book *Taqwim al Abdan* by Ibn Jazlah, 11th century A.D.

Name of the disease Aspects	AL SADR (Confusion & dizziness)	AL DAWAR (Vertigo)	AL SARAA (Epilepsy)	AL SAKTA (Stroke)	AL KABOOS (Nightmare)	AL MALIKHOULIA & AL MARAQIYAH (Melancholia and hypochondria, ?obsession)	AL QATARAT (?Insanity)	AL ISHQ (Love sickness)
Treatment or constitution	cold and humid	cold	cold	cold	cold	dry	dry	hot
Age	elderly	elderly	children & adolescents	elderly	elderly	very old and young	very old and young	young
Season	winter	winter	winter	winter	winter	autumn	autumn and winter	all seasons seasons
Country favorable for disease	cold and humid	cold	cold	cold	cold	dry	dry	more in the east
Prognosis	dangerous at extremes	not dangerous	dangerous if frequent	dangerous	not dangerous	dangerous	dangerous	not dangerous
Causes								
Symptoms								
Blood letting, vomiting, etc.								
Royal treatment								
Common treatment								

Table 1. Translation of table of mental illnesses, their description and their treatment from the book *Taqwim al Abdan* by Ibn Jazlah, 11th century A.D. The last five lines have not been translated—see the original table.

Some Continuing Arabic Medical Traditions

Apart from nomenclature and classification, there are many traditions of Arabic medicine which have become integral parts of medical thinking of the people in countries in which the influence of Islamic medicine was strong. This is particularly true of India and Pakistan. The following examples may be illustrative:

1) *Diagnosis by examination of the pulse:* The Arabic physicians had a tradition of diagnosing the disease mainly by examining the pulse of the patient. Many patients in Pakistan and India would begin the interview by offering their wrist for examination and feel a little disappointed if the doctor does not pay attention to the pulse.

2) *The concept of "hot" and "cold" foods:* These concepts are very central to the Arabic materia medica and therapeutic principles. For example, each food article is supposed to have a special property of having a "hot" or "cold" or "moist" and "dry" effect on the body. It is not conceived in terms of physical temperature, rather its supposed effect is on metabolism. The human temperament, diseases, herbal medicines, etc., are all divided on such principles. For example, a patient may tell the doctor that "I hope your medicine is not 'hot' type because that may not suit my system."

3) *The concept of "Perhez":* At the end of a medical interview, the patient would generally ask the doctor about *perhez* or what type of food or behavior one should avoid for quick recovery. Even in the modern medical practice such an approach offers a very good opportunity for health education.

Psychiatric Aspects of Traditional Chinese Medicine

For an outsider, the system of traditional medicine of China is very complex. Like other ancient systems of medicine, it is intimately linked with the prevailing religious and philosophical thought, which is difficult to grasp by one unfamiliar with Chinese culture. It is generally accepted that, historically, the main core of Chinese medicine separated itself from magico-religious concepts of diseases earlier than in other cultures (Needham & Lu Gwei-Djen, 1969).

The three major religious philosophies in Chinese culture have been Taosim, Buddhism and Confucianism. According to Mora (1980), the following is true:

Regardless of particular school of thought and emphasis, the old Chinese concepts of humans and universe center on three main tenets: (1) the world was not created by a divine, supernatural being but by TAO, an abstract principle that turned into an active moral guide after creation was accomplished, (2) Humans are composed of the same elements of the universe and reflect in themselves the principles of the macrocosm, (3) Mental functions are not conceived distinct from physical function and are not localized in any part of the organism though the heart is given particular importance as a guide for the mind.

Another very central concept in Chinese tradition is that of the Yin and Yang as two parts, in a perennial state of opposition and attraction.

One of the source books of Chinese medicine is the *Canon of Internal Medicine* (Nei Jing) which dates back to the 4th century B.C. and has subsequently been brought up in numerous editions (Chinese Medicine, 1987). It refers to mental disorders like insanity, dementia, violent behavior and convulsions (Mora, 1980). Possession by spirits was also recognized. In the field of treatment, the most important contribution of Chinese medicine has been that of acupuncture, which has retained its popularity up to modern times.

Medical Traditions in Africa

While the northern part of Africa came greatly under the influence of Muslim empires, Sub-Saharan Africa remained largely free of the influence of other civilizations till the arrival of European colonial powers in the 18th century or so. Though there were at times large powerful African empires like the Masai of East Africa, African society largely remained divided into various tribes, each one having its separate traditions and culture.

It is generally accepted that the dominant feature of traditional medicine in Africa has been the beliefs in gods, spirits of ancestors and supernatural powers. In many parts of Africa nearly all forms of illness, personal catastrophes, accidents, and unusual happenings were generally attributed to machinations of the enemy and malicious influence of spirits that inhabit the world around, though according to Lambo this is not the whole story (Lambo, 1969). Many of the tribes were also aware of the concept of the natural causation. This was particularly true of Masai tribe of East Africa and the Shona tribe of present-day Zimbabwe. According to Swift and Asuni (1975), the Shona people identify four general causes of mental illness, which is diagnosed when a person does not talk sense or behaves in a strange or foolish manner. Such a person may be restless, violent or very quiet. These four causes are the influence of the spirits, old age, worry or guilt for a wrong or immoral act, and the improper development of the brain (Swift & Asuni, 1975).

Prince (1964), who surveyed 46 traditional healers among the Yoruba, identified three large groups of factors believed to cause disease and other misfortune:

1) Natural causes like bad blood, bad odor, smoking cannabis, hereditary factors.

2) Magical influence resulting from witchcraft and curses.

3) God sending spirits to punish those who have offended him.

Yoruba healers considered roughly half the mental diseases they see
as being due to magical causes. However, it must be emphasized that
there is not a uniform pattern, and such views vary from one tribal
group to another (Swift & Asuni, 1975). This was particularly evident
in the study of psychosis in four East African tribes from Uganda,
Kenya and Tanzania (Edgerton, 1966).

It is sometimes said that medical thought in Africa is "prelogical" in
contrast to Western industrial societies, where the medical science is
"logical." This may not necessarily be so. As Tigani Mahi pointed out,
"magic has its own order of logic and reason." In a similar vein, Lambo
has remarked that the African mind is not prelogical, rather it is a
"possessor of a type of knowledge that teaches that reality consists in
the relation not of men with things but of men with other men and of
all men with spirits" (Lambo, 1969).

Conceptual Differences Between Traditional and Modern Systems of Medicine in Psychiatric Diagnosis and Classification

1) The etiology of most of the mental disorders is still unknown. In the
   Third World, magico-religious traditions still persist in many countries, particularly in the rural societies. As a result, many varieties of
   psychotic, neurotic and personality disorders are understood by the
   general population as being the result of spirit possession or witchcraft. However, if the patient consults a practitioner of well-organ-
   ized traditional medical systems like Ayurveda, Chinese or Islamic
   medicine, the explanation provided is usually on the lines of "scientific" theory of that system, e.g., imbalance of body humours, etc.

2) In the European philosophical tradition there is a strong tendency to
   think in terms of duality or "polarity of contrasting opposites" (Wig,
   1985; Mora, 1980). In modern psychiatry this has often led to an
   undue preoccupation with controversies like nature/nurture,
   body/mind, conscious/unconscious, organic/functional and so on.
   This has also influenced modern psychiatric classifications. Other
   cultures have looked at the nature differently, often "by juxtaposition
   and identification of polarities" (Mora, 1980). The Chinese theory of

Yin-Yang principles is a beautiful example of this. In Indian philosophy, instead of two models, there are often three dimensions of a phenomenon, e.g., the Tri-Guna theory of inherent qualities of nature as *sattva*, *rajas* and *tamas* or Triumverate of Gods, Brahma, Vishnu and Shiva controlling three aspects of creation, preservation and destruction of the universe.

3) The concept of insanity as a grossly disturbed behavior with loss of insight seems to be well recognized in most of the ancient medical texts. However, such a diagnosis was based predominantly on observation of external behavior. The intrapsychic processes as such were neither given prominence nor used as basis of diagnosis or classification. For example, in Indian Ayurvedic texts there is no clear recognition of separate affective or mood disorders, nor is there any clear description of insanity resembling paranoid psychosis, while states of excitement, severe withdrawal and socially inappropriate behavior are well described. The common people in the Third-World countries, including health workers and auxiliaries, easily recognize conditions like acute or chronic psychosis as clear examples of mental illness, but conditions like depression, hypomania and paranoid state are less easily accepted as medical or psychiatric problems.

4) The current division of functional psychoses into affective disorders and schizophrenia seem to be based on the 19th century European understanding of human mind into arbitrary divisions of "feeling" and "thinking." Such concepts do not find a recognition in traditional Third-World classifications.

5) Unlike modern medicine as it is practiced in many sites today, the traditional systems of medicine do not maintain a strict division between body and mind. For example, the imbalance between body humours can affect both the physical as well as mental functions. As a result, the practitioners of traditional medical systems tend to have a more holistic approach toward their patients. A traditional practitioner does not use the modern medical approach of excluding the organic illness before thinking of psychological causes. Furthermore, a neurotic patient feels more comfortable with a traditional healer because there is no tendency to be labeled as having no "physical" illness and hence to be considered psychologically "inferior," as is common in predominantly biologically oriented practitioners of modern medicine.

6) The concept of "subconscious" processes is relatively new in modern psychiatry. It has no roots in the Third-World traditions. In modern psychiatric classification this has often led to the assumption of "underlying" illness in the absence of overt manifestations. Subconscious processes were also seen as the underlying cause for illnesses

such as hysteria and somatoform disorders. In the Third World, lay persons as well as nonspecialist doctors and health workers find such reasoning often difficult to comprehend.

7) In the traditional medical systems there is no unified concept of neurosis as has emerged in the modern psychiatry during the last 100 years. Though feelings of fear and grief are recognized by all cultures, only in modern medicine has an excess of these types of emotion been given the status of medical diseases like anxiety and depression. An excess of all emotions has been considered harmful in all cultures, but modern psychiatry has chosen only two of them as "disorders." It is difficult to explain why, if an excess of anxiety or depression is a disease, an excess of hate or anger or greed or lust should *not* be regarded as pathological.

8) The classification of personality types and personality disorders has received considerable attention in the traditional medical systems. In general, the classification of personality was closely modeled on the prevailing religious and moral codes of human behavior. It is uncertain whether the diagnosis of personality disorder can be made by reference to the observer's own value system. A major difference in the classification of personality disorders in the traditional medical literature and in the modern psychiatry is that while the modern psychiatry uses the concept of average norm, i.e., whatever is markedly deviant is abnormal, the traditional medical systems of the Third World prefer the ideal norm, i.e., whatever is less than ideal is inadequate and thus, in a sense, abnormal.

9) The modern psychiatric concept of personality disorders gives the impression that maladaptive patterns of behavior are nearly permanent and not amenable to improvement in any significant way. This is especially so in the case of antisocial personality. However, many non-European cultures do not emotionally react in this manner to the concept of personality disorders. As depicted in the old Indian epics and the present-day Indian film stories, in popular imagination a bad person can often turn good under a strong emotional impact. Even in present times, many Muslims, under the impact of pilgrimage to holy Mecca, are able to change their personality and give up vices like drug dependence.

The Use of Modern Psychiatric Classifications in the Third World Countries

In spite of considerable popularity of the traditional medical systems in many countries, the bulk of the health services including psychiatric services which have evolved in the countries of the Third World are largely based on the modern medical system. Despite the dissatisfaction with many aspects of international classification of diseases, most of the countries fully recognize the importance and utility of a universally acceptable classification. In fact, many developing countries have been rendering full support to the WHO for the development of such an international psychiatric classification.

In some developing countries (e.g., India, Egypt, Indonesia) efforts have been made in recent years to develop "national" classifications of psychiatric disorders (Wig & Singh, 1967; Shaheen, 1985; Okasha, 1988). Most of the time, such efforts are in keeping with the existing international classifications; English, American, and French textbooks of psychiatry are used in many countries and have also influenced these national efforts. The recent developments in American psychiatry leading to the emergence of the *Diagnostic and Statistical Manual, Third Edition* (DSM-III) has particularly impressed the psychiatrists in the developing countries by its empirical approach and provision of diagnostic criteria. However, DSM-III has many limitations for the needs of the Third-World countries (Wig, 1983), which wish to use an improved but common international classification.

It should also be kept in mind that, for the majority of the routine psychiatric services in the developing countries, there are only a limited number of diagnostic categories that are regularly and frequently used. Hence, the academic disputes between different psychiatric schools regarding the correctness of labeling for a rare syndrome is of limited importance from the point of view of public health services.

A recent survey done in India is illustrative of this point (Kala, 1985). A questionnaire was sent to psychiatric units in 112 general hospitals and 24 mental hospitals regarding the use of ICD 9 during the year 1983. Thirty-eight respondents from general hospitals and ten from mental hospitals replied. In all 116,430 psychiatric patients were seen in these services during the year. Almost all respondents considered the International Classification of Diseases (ICD 9) as "mostly suitable" for their needs. None of them felt that ICD 9 is "useless" or "unsuitable for the majority of cases." Four diagnostic categories of ICD 9, i.e., 296 (affective psychoses), 295 (schizophrenia), 300 (neurotic disorders), and 298 (other nonorganic psychosis) covered 85% of all cases seen. Organic psychoses, 290-94, and mental retardation, 317-19, added another 5% to this figure. Some of the least used categories (used less than one in a 1000 cases) were 305 (nondependent use of drugs), 302 (sexual deviations and disorders), and 297 (paranoid states). Less frequently used categories included 301 (personality disorders), 308 (acute reaction to stress), and 311 (depressive reactions not elsewhere classified). Eighteen respondents out of 48 (37%) felt that there is need for an additional category of "acute psychosis" not well covered at present under categories 295, 296 or 298.

Shortcomings of Contemporary Psychiatric Classification as Applied to Countries of the Third World

Medical and psychiatric professionals in the countries of the Third World have expressed dissatisfaction with the contemporary psychiatric classifications from time to time in various international forums (Wig et al., 1985). Most of this criticism has been directed toward the traditional European and American classifications, which are part of every standard textbook on psychiatry, and which have formed the basis of training for most of the medical and psychiatric specialists in the countries of the Third World. It was generally felt that these classifications neither reflect the reality of psychiatric phenomenology as seen in the Third World nor meet the needs of its growing health services. During the last 20 years, the World Health Organization has tried to rectify this situation by encouraging greater input from experts from developing countries in various WHO expert panels on classification. This was reflected in drafting the eighth and ninth revisions of the ICD, but a much stronger involvement of Third-World experts was sought for the development of a classification of mental disorder in the 10th edition of the ICD, which is currently in the process of being finalized. A recent publication (Sartorius, 1988) discussed various issues related to psychiatric classification and listed over 150 experts from all parts of the world, including many from the countries of the Third World, who participated in these discussions. Many more experts, however, were involved: The field tests of the new revision have been carried out in many languages in some 190 centers located in 55 different countries.

The criticism of contemporary psychiatric classification by psychiatrists of the Third-World countries is usually based on cultural grounds, health services and on clinical grounds.

Shortcomings of Current Classificatory Systems Related to Cultural Differences

As has been pointed out above, contemporary psychiatric diagnosis and classification have evolved in Europe and North America only during the last 100 years and reflect the style of thinking and cultural bias of that society. In the countries of the Third World, most of which have only recently attained political independence, there is a legitimate feeling of national and regional cultural pride. Many of these countries are inheritors of some of the world's oldest civilizations, with well-developed traditional systems of medicines which are still serving a large part of their populations. Mental health professionals working in these countries often find themselves in a difficult position, divided between the loyalty to modern scientific knowledge in which they have been educated and loyalty to traditional cultural values in which they have been brought up since childhood. Many of their patients and members of health staff share the psychological concepts described in the traditional medical systems but which are insufficient to accommodate the growing knowledge in psychiatry or the complex needs of the modern health services.

One example of this kind of cultural criticism is the exaggerated space and importance contemporary psychiatric classification gives to disorders commonly seen in European or North American settings, but which are not common in Asia, Africa and Latin America, for example, eating disorders, like anorexia nervosa or bulimia, phobic and panic disorders, sexual deviations and personality disorders. In contrast, many conditions that are relatively common in the Third-World countries find only a cursory mention in contemporary classifications, e.g,. acute psychotic disorders, hysterical symptoms, phenomena of spirit possession and multiple somatization disorders.

Many observers have stressed that patients in developing countries express themselves more easily in somatic than in psychological terms. As a result of this, many subcategories in European and American classifications based on the presence of symptoms related to the patient's complaint are difficult to apply in the countries of the Third World.

Shortcomings on Health Services Grounds

It is being increasingly recognized in the countries of the Third World that a large number of mental health problems do not reach a psychiatrist and are being cared for by nonspecialists. The highly insufficient psychiatrist-to-population ratio in developing countries makes it necessary that even severe mental disorders be treated by nonpsychiatrists. Furthermore, with the recent emphasis on incorporation of psychiatric services into primary health care, primary-care-level workers and physicians are increasingly using psychiatric diagnoses. The existing classifications are obviously too complex for such use.

It is thus necessary that a parallel, management-oriented, simple psychiatric classification for use at the primary level be prepared. Some attempts have already been made in this direction. One recent WHO study (Sartorius & Harding, 1983), which was simultaneously carried out in the countries of Brazil, Columbia, Egypt, India, Philippines, Senegal and Sudan, brought out the need for simplified psychiatric diagnostic procedures and training programs for primary-care doctors and health workers in these countries. In India, Srinivasa Murthy and Wig (1983) found that, for the training of health workers, simplified concepts of acute and chronic psychosis, severe depression, epilepsy and mental retardation were easy to put across and were meaningful in terms of management. In recent years, primary-care health personnel in a number of countries in the Eastern Mediterranean Region and Southeast Asia have received mental health training using a limited number of diagnostic conditions (WHO/EMRO, 1988).

Shortcomings on Clinical Grounds

In the absence of knowledge about the etiology of most of the mental disorders, contemporary psychiatric classifications are far from perfect. Boundaries are difficult to draw between one disorder and the other. All the major syndromes, like anxiety and depression, schizophrenia and affective psychoses, imperceptibly merge into each other. Psychiatrists in the Third World share all these clinical problems with their colleagues in Europe and North American. However, in their clinical work, they have additional problems resulting from the differences in the type of disorders they see in their practice in developing countries.

The number of psychiatrists in the countries of the Third World has grown rapidly during the last three decades. In India, where there were less than 50 qualified psychiatrists at the time of independence in 1947, there are now more than 2000 psychiatrists. There has been a similar rapid increase in other developing countries like Indonesia, Pakistan, Iran, Egypt, Nigeria, Sudan, etc. This has been mainly due to the development of university departments of psychiatry with facilities for postgraduate training. These departments have also stimulated better record keeping and research. As a result of this, considerable data has accumulated about psychiatric symptomatology and diagnostic practices in the countries of the Third World, which could greatly help in improving psychiatric classifications. Unfortunately, a large part of such material remains unpublished; and when published results are presented in national/medical journals or in local languages, it works against their wide distribution and visibility.

On the basis of review of such literature and on the basis of personal experience of the author, the following diagnostic areas in the current systems of classification are pointed out where specific difficulties are experienced by the psychiatrists in the Third World:

1) *Organic mental disorders:* Classification of "functional" psychotic disorders that appear in the background of systemic infections, malnutrition, head injury, epilepsy, etc.

2) *Psychotic disorders:* Acute and transient psychotic disorders that do not clearly fit into either schizophrenia or affective psychosis.

3) *Neurotic disorders:* (a) Multiple somatic symptoms without demonstrable physical pathology; (b) Classification of hysterical symptoms.

4) *"Culture-bound" syndromes:* Classification of "folk illnesses" or culture-bound symptoms like *koro, latah, amok,* various types of spirit possession states, culture-bound sexual symptoms, e.g., Dhat syndrome, etc.

5) *Classification of personality disorders, sexual deviations, drug dependence, childhood psychiatric disorders.*

Specialists in these clinical fields are relatively few in the countries of the Third World, and clinical data that could help in improving the fit between the classifications and the patients' problems are still scarce.

Organic Mental Disorders

In the countries of the Third World, organic conditions, like malnourishment, cerebral and systemic infections, epilepsy, etc., are still widely prevalent. Hence, it is quite common to see different kinds of acute and chronic organic mental disorders especially in general hospital psychiatry. The difficulty of diagnosis and classification is experienced particularly in the following two situations:

1) Although it is possible to make a syndromic diagnosis "organic" disorder, it is often difficult to ascribe it to a simple cause of the organic disorder because more than one causal factor (infection, malnutrition, injury or epilepsy) is often present. Even when this is not the case, the lack of adequate modern investigative facilities in most centers makes it difficult to decide on the etiological assignation of cases seen in clinical practice.

2) There are a number of cases who present with prominent functional psychotic symptoms (e.g., excitement, stupor, hallucinations, delusions, catatonia) who also have high fever or are suffering from infectious (or other) diseases. These cases often receive labels like "typhoid psychosis" or "malaria psychosis" rather than the diagnosis of, say, schizophrenia, which would have been warranted by the symptoms seen in the patient. There is a similar problem in classifying psychotic symptoms occurring in people with epilepsy, which are quite common in Africa and Asia (Asuni & Pillutla, 1967; Shukla et al., 1979).

In this respect, the proposed draft of the ICD 10 is a distinct improvement over previous psychiatric classifications. It offers the psychiatrist a choice of a wide range of psychiatric clinical syndromes like organic anxiety state, depressive state, hallucinosis, catatonia, or schizophrenia-like state, etc., which can be made even if the etiology of the organic mental disorder is not known. The ICD allows, of course, that the underlying cause be stated and classified.

Acute and Transient Psychotic Disorders

The concept of temporary insanity has been recognized in the medical literature for a long time. Following Kraepelin's broad division of functional psychosis into dementia praecox and manic depressive psychosis, the interest in these acute transient disorders seems to have been temporarily reduced, especially in British and German psychiatry. In French psychiatry, the traditional separation between acute and chronic type of psychotic symptoms has persisted and a variety of diagnostic choices are offered to the psychiatrist (Ey, 1954; Stengel, 1959). In the Scandinavian countries, a tradition of making the diagnosis of reactive or psychogenic psychosis has received prominence and remained a point of controversy in most efforts to agree on a uniform system of psychiatric classification.

In the countries of the Third World, the modern psychiatric traditions have generally followed the tradition of the training center of the European host country where the local psychiatrists have received their training. For example, countries like India, Pakistan, Sudan and Nigeria have followed the British psychiatric tradition, while Senegal, Tunisia and Morocco have followed the French psychiatric tradition of diagnosis and classification. Lately, many of these countries have also been influenced by the developments in American psychiatry.

From the point of view of a psychiatrist practicing in a Third World country, the following issues are of particular importance for the classification of acute psychotic disorders:

1) Numerous reports from Asia and Africa and Latin America suggest that these disorders are relatively common in developing countries (Wig et al., 1985). According to German (1972), the "presence of amorphous, easily precipitated and recurrent transient psychosis is one of the main differences in clinical psychiatry in Africa from psychiatry in other parts of the world." A recent WHO multinational study (to be published) on acute psychosis confirmed the high prevalence of such disorders among hospital admissions in the Philippines, India, Sudan, Senegal, Columbia, Cuba and other countries. In a recently completed multicentred Indian study sponsored by the Indian Council of Medical Research, it was found that acute psychosis—symptoms appearing acutely and becoming full-blown psychosis within two weeks—constituted more than 10% of all psychosis cases seen in these centers. The percentage will be much higher in patients 15–30 years old (ICMR Report, 1986).

2) A large number of cases of acute psychotic disorders are difficult to fit into the traditional categories of schizophrenia or affective psychosis. In the Indian Council of Medical Research (ICMR) study, the number of fresh onset cases that could not be fitted into ICD 9 categories of schizophrenia and affective psychosis was over 40%. Using the "CATEGO" program, only 20% of the cases were labeled as definite schizophrenia, 19% as definite manic depressive psychosis and 6% as depressive psychosis. Of the remaining 55%, 35% could not be classified into any clear-cut diagnostic category, while another 20% were assigned to more than one CATEGO class (ICMR Report, 1986).

3) Many studies in all parts of the world have pointed out the good outcome in these acute psychotic disorders. In the above-mentioned ICMR study, the full recovery at the end of one year was 75–85%.

4) Though psychological stress seem to be related to acute psychotic disorders, it is not present in all the cases. In a number of recent Indian studies, it seems that only about half the cases have a stressful life event or somatic or physiological stress immediately preceding the acute psychotic disorders (ICMR Report, 1986; Wig & Parhee, 1984; Kapur & Pandurangi, 1979; Singh & Sachdev, 1980).

The proper recognition and classification of acute and transient psychotic disorders requires particular attention at this point in time. These disorders are frequent and of major public health importance. They cannot be classified with either schizophrenia or affective disorders. Many of the cases are not "reactive," i.e., related to some recent life event. The terms like "schizophreniform" might force us to think in terms of a schizophrenic illness, which is not necessary. Criteria of a chronic disabling disease should not be applied to an acute and transient disorder. Genetic studies may ultimately clarify whether these disorders have a link with schizophrenic or affective disorders, but for the time being we must keep our mind open. The effectiveness of dopamine blockade agents in all functional psychotic symptoms (schizophrenia, mania or acute psychotic disorders) also throws doubt on the current divisions among functional psychosis (Johnstone et al., 1988). More research particularly on the long-term development of acute psychotic disorders in the countries of the Third World is highly desirable.

The new draft of ICD 10 is a great advance over previous classifications. It not only recognizes the presence of such acute and transient psychotic disorders but further groups them into convenient subgroups on the basis of available knowledge as follows:

— F23.0 Acute polymorphic psychotic disorder (without symptoms of schizophrenia)

— F23.1 Acute polymorphic psychotic disorder with symptoms of schizophrenia

— F23.2 Acute schizophrenia-like psychotic disorder

— F23.3 Other acute predominantly delusional psychotic episode

— F23.8 Other acute and transient psychotic episode.

A 5th or 6th character (4th or 5th digit) can be used to indicate whether or not the acute psychotic disorder is associated with acute stress or had an abrupt onset.

Culture-Bound Syndromes

This somewhat unfortunate term has come to denote a heterogeneous group of disorders that have only one thing in common: they occur in cultures other than those prevailing in the USA and Western Europe and do not easily fit into the system of psychiatric diagnosis and classification developed in these countries. Since Kraepelin's visit to Indonesia nearly 100 years ago, there has been great interest in these syndromes by many psychiatrists and anthropologists. Recently, a comprehensive book on the subject of culture-bound syndromes was published (Simons & Hughes, 1985). It contains an excellent glossary of almost all the currently known culture-bound or folk psychiatric syndromes.

There is a common debate among psychiatrists in the Third-World countries regarding the place of the culture-bound syndromes in modern psychiatric classification. Some have favored grouping them separately, while others have favored amalgamating them in existing rubrics of psychiatric classification. In the view of the present author, it would be better to accommodate various culture-bound syndromes into the existing international classification, which foresees the possibility of having separate codes for national needs. Culture influences all aspects of health and illness, and it thus affects all psychiatric syndromes. It is likely that there will be cultural differences in the clinical presentation of a case suffering from anxiety or depression or schizophrenia, as seen in England, China or Nigeria. The stronger the roots of patients in their culture, the more likely such variations become. Therefore, it seems artificial to separate out a few conditions like *koro*, *latah* or *amok* for special consideration as culture-bound syndromes. Though these culture-bound syndromes are of great academic interest for our understanding of the role of culture and illness, from the public health point of view, the crucial questions are how common such culture bound symptoms are in the existing health services of a country. Will their separation into separate diagnostic categories help in the better management of these cases in the country health services? Judged by these criteria, there are relatively few conditions that require separate coding.

It is not in the interest of the psychiatrists from Third-World countries to demand the separation of all culture-bound syndromes into a separate classification group. It will only tend to increase the isolation of Third-World psychiatry. It is more important, however, whenever such a condition is considered necessary for separation by a national group, that it should be possible to do so within the existing frame work of the international classification. The national and international classifications should, however, at all times remain translatable one into another.

The new draft of the ICD 10 provides an adequate scope for such groupings. Most of the culture-bound symptoms can be classified under the standard diagnostic groups of organic mental disorders, acute psychotic disorders or neurotic and stress-related disorders.

Neurotic and Stress-Related Disorders

The use of the term neurosis has led to great dissatisfaction in the countries of the Third World. The concept of subconscious mental forces and intrapsychic processes has not been very easily acceptable to most of the patients as well the clinicians in the developing countries. It leads to a biased perception of the patient's problems. The term "anxiety neurosis" (or "anxiety state" as in ICD 9) is used frequently but not very specifically in the Third-World countries. However, only a few cases present with acute anxiety episodes or sufficiently clear psychological or physiological manifestations of anxiety. A large number of patients who get the label of "anxiety neurosis" actually present with multiple somatic symptoms and vague aches and pains, underlying anxiety being presumed by the psychiatrists.

Hysterical symptoms, though reported to be rare now in Europe and USA, continue to be a common presentation in the general health services in the developing world. The current subclassification of hysterical symptoms, however, is unsatisfactory. The classical division into conversion and dissociation or between motor or sensory symptoms is arbitrary, unsatisfactory and artificial. Hysterical fits, one of the commonest presentations of hysteria in developing countries, are really a combination of conversion and dissociation (Saxena, 1987). The distinction between conversion and dissociation, moreover, does not help in predicting outcome. It may be more useful to distinguish between acute hysterical reactions and chronic hysterical symptoms, both for management and prognosis (Wig et al., 1982).

Numerous psychiatrists in developing countries have repeatedly observed that among the most common presentation in the psychiatric services at the primary care level are cases with multiple somatic symptoms without structural pathology. Depending on the inclination and training of the clinician, these cases are currently labeled as chronic anxiety, hysteria, neurotic depression, neurasthenia or hypochondriasis. The introduction of the term "somatoform disorders" in the American DSM-III has improved the classification in this area. The new draft of the ICD 10 is a further improvement. It has grouped the Somatoform disorders in the following subgrouping:

— Somatization disorder

— Undifferentiated somatoform disorder

— Hypochondriacal disorder

— Somatoform autonomic dysfunction

— Persistent pain disorder

This grouping is likely to be useful in the developing countries.

Conclusions

1) The psychiatrists in the Third-World countries find themselves in a difficult position in the matter of psychiatric diagnosis and classification. The psychological concepts and psychiatric nomenclature prevalent in the traditional systems of medicine, though still popular with the lay public and many health professionals, are insufficient to accommodate the growing knowledge in psychiatry or the complex health needs of the modern health services. On the other hand, a total

switch to a European or American classification proves equally frustrating.

2) Recognizing the need for an international consensus, psychiatrists in the Third World have generally supported the international classification of diseases. However, they were not fully satisfied with it because it had to make concessions to various disparate—in the past mainly European and American—schools of thought, which often make the international classification too elaborate and weakens its logical structure. In order to bring the best solution to the problems of classification, the ICD has to be suitably modified to serve the need of the countries in the Third World. The current effort of the WHO to involve a large number of psychiatrists from many countries in the development of the 10th Revision of the ICD are most welcome and are likely to result in a vastly improved classification.

3) Psychiatrists in the Third World are impressed by certain phenomena that cannot be satisfactorily classified in the current classifications. Two important examples are, first, the category of "acute psychotic disorders" as an entity distinct from schizophrenia and affective psychosis and, second, the large number of cases of somatic complaints without physical basis that do not clearly fall into any well-defined "neurosis." Enough data are now available in the countries of the Third World to justify a fresh look at the classification of these disorders.

4) With the increasing use of psychiatric diagnosis by nonspecialists and the rapid development of community psychiatric services, it is necessary that a parallel, simple, management-oriented classification be prepared for use at the primary health care level.

5) The new draft of the ICD 10 is a great advance in the field of psychiatric diagnosis and classification. It does not subscribe to any one national school and has attempted to accommodate most of the needs of the countries of the Third World. There are still large areas, like the classification of hysteria, of personality disorders and child psychiatric disorders, that do not satisfy the mental health professionals in the Third World. Changing these parts of the classification, however, is only possible if more data are generated and research undertaken in the field of psychiatric diagnosis and classification in the countries of the Third World.

Acknowledgement

I am grateful to Dr Khayat of WHO/EMRO for his help in the translation of many relevant Arabic medical texts consulted for this paper and his general advice about writing of the section on Arabic Medicine. I would also like to express my sincere thanks to Dr Sartorius of the WHO, Geneva, for his helpful criticism and editorial revision of this paper.

References

Asuni, T. and Pillutla, V.S. Schizophrenia like psychosis in Nigerian epileptics. *Brit J Psychiat* 113, 1375-1379 (1967).

Baasher, T., The Arab countries. In: Howells J.G. (Ed.) *World History of Psychiatry*. London: Bailliere and Tindall, 547–578 (1975).

Balodhi, J.P. Constituting the outlines of a philosophy of Ayurveda—Mainly on mental health import. *Ind J. Psychiatry* 29(2) 127–131 (1987).

Chinese Medicine. *What is New in China Series* (18). China Reconstructs Press. Beijing (1987).

Deb Sikdar, B.M. Glimpses of medico-psychological practices in ancient India. *Ind J. Psychiat* 111(4), 250–259 (1961).

Dube, K.C. Nosology and therapy of mental illness in Ayurveda. *Comparative Medicine East and West* VI, 3, 209–228 (1978).

Edgerton, R.B. Conception of psychosis in four East African societies. *American Anthropologist* 68(2) Part I, 408–425 (1966).

Ey, H. Les problemes cliniques des schizophrenics. *Evol Psychiatry* 149: 212, 94–101 (1954).

German, G.A. Aspects of clinical psychiatry in Sub-Saharan Africa. *Brit J Psychiat* 121, 461–79 (1972).

Graziani, J.S. *Arabic medicine in the eleventh century as represented in the works of Ibn Jazlah*. Hamdard Academy, Karachi, Pakistan (1980).

Haly Abbas (also spelled as Ali Abbas) Kamel Al-Sina'ah (Liber Regius), Dar Al-Tiba'a Press, Cairo, 1889 A.D. (original in Arabic).

Indian Council of Medical Research. *The phenomenology and natural history of acute psychosis: Report of a collaborative study at Bikaner, Goa, Patiala, Vellore*. Mimeographed report. Published by Indian Council of Medical Research, New Delhi 160029, India (1986).

Johnstone, E.C., Crow, T.J., Frith, C.D., Owens, D.G. The Northwick-Park "Functional" Psychosis Study. Diagnosis and treatment response. *The Lancet* 119–125 (1988).

Jolly, J. *Indian Medicine* (Translated from the German and supplemented with notes by Kashikar, C.G.). New Delhi: Munshiram Manoharlal Publishers Pvt Ltd. (1977).

Kala, A.K. Utility of ICD-9 for Indian patients: An opinion survey. *Ind J Psychiat* 27(3), 253–254 (1985).

Kapur, R.L. and Pandurangi, A.K. A comparative study of reactive psychosis and acute psychosis without precipitating stress. *Brit J Psychiat* 135, 544–550 (1979).

Khayat, M.H. *The history of clinical chemistry in Arab-Islamic medicine*. Paper presented at the World Congress of Clinical Chemistry, Vienna (1981).

Lambo, T.A. Traditional African cultures and Western medicine: A critical review. In: Poynter, F.N.L. (Ed.) *Culture and medicine*. London. Welcome Institute of the History of Medicine (1969).

Mora, G. Historical and theoretical trends in psychiatry. In: Kaplan H.I., Freedman, A.M., Sadock, B.J. (Eds.) *Comprehensive textbook of psychiatry/III, Volume I.* 4–98 (1980).

Narayana Reddy, G.N., Ramu, M.G. and Venkataram, B.S. Concept of manas (Psyche) in Ayurveda. *NIMHANS Journal* 5(2), 125–131 (1987).

Needam, J. and Lu Gwei-Djen. Chinese medicine: In Poynter, F.N.L. (Ed.) *Medicine and culture*. London. Welcome Institute of History of Medicine (1969).

Okasha, A. *Clinical psychiatry*. The Anglo Egyptian Bookshop, Cairo (1988).

Prince, R. Indigenous Yoruba psychiatry. In: Kiev, A. (Ed.) *Magic, faith and healing.* London, Collier-Macmillan (1964).

Ramu, M.G., Venkataram, B.S., Janakiramaiah, N. Manovikaras with special reference to Udvega (anxiety) and Vishad (depression). *NIMHANS Journal* 6(1), 41–46 (1988).

Rao, K.N., Medical manpower: Needs for a comprehensive health care in India. *Ind. J. Med. Education* April 1966, Vol. 3, (quoted by N.H. Keswani in Poynter FNL (Ed.) *Medicine and culture*. London, Welcome Institute of History of Medicine, 1969).

Samarqandi Najeebuddin. *Aetiology, causes, signs and symptomatology*. A manuscript from around 1400 A.D. (original in Arabic). (Personal communication from Dr Khayat).

Sartorius, N. International perspectives of psychiatric classification. *Brit J of Psychiat* 152 (suppl. I) 9–14 (1988).

Sartorius, N. and Harding, T.W. The WHO collaborative study on strategies for extension of mental health care. I. The genesis of the study. *Am J Psychiat* 140: 11, 1470–1473 (1983).

Saxena, S. "Simple Dissociative Disorder." A Subcategory in DSM III R (Letter to Editor). *Am J Psychiat* 144: 4, 524–525 (1987).

Shaheen, O. *Diagnostic criteria of psychiatric disorders: A comparative study*. Department of Psychiatry, Cairo University (1985).

Shukla, G.D., Srivastva, O.N., Katiyar, B.C., Joshi, V. and Mohan, P.K. Psychiatric manifestations of temporal lobe epilepsy: A controlled study. *Brit J Psychiat* 135, 411 (1979).

Simons, R.C. and Hughes, C.C. *The culture-bound syndromes: Folk illnesses of psychiatric and anthropological interest*. D. Reidel Publishing Co. Dordrecht/Boston (1985).

Singh, G. and Sachdev, J.S. A clinical and follow up study of atypical psychosis. *Ind J Psychiat* 22, 167–72.

Srinivasa Murthy, R. and Wig, N. The WHO collaborative study on strategies for extending mental health care, IV: A training approach to enhancing the availability of mental health manpower in a developing country. *Am J Psychiat* 140: 11, 1486–1490 (1983).

Stengel, E. Classification of mental disorders. *Bull WHO* 21, 601–663 (1959).

Swift, C.R. and Asuni, T. *Mental health and disease in Africa*. Churchill Livingstone (1975).

Varma, L.P. Psychiatry in Ayurveda. *Ind. J. Psychiat*. VII(4), 292–312 (1965).

Weiss, M.G. *Critical study of Unmada (Insanity) in the early Sanskrit medical literature: An Analysis of Ayurvedic psychiatry with reference to the present day diagnostic categories*. University of Pennsylvania. Ph.D., dissertation in South East Asia Regional studies. Ann Arbor University Microfilms (1977).

WHO/EMRO. Intercountry workshop on training in mental health in primary health care. Islamabad, 7–12 March 1987. EM/MENT/114-E. WHO Regional Office for the Eastern Mediterranean Region, Alexandria (1988).

Wig, N.N. Psychiatric classification—A view from the Third World. In Pichot, P., Berner, P., Wolf, R. and Thau K. (Eds.) *Psychiatry—The state of the art, Vol. I. Clinical psychopathology, nomenclature and classification*. New York, Plenum Press, 45–50 (1985).

Wig, N.N. DSM III—Its strengths and weaknesses: A perspective from the Third World. In: Spitzer, R.L., Williams I.B.W. and Skodol, A.E. (Eds.) *International perspective on DSM III*. American Psychiatric Press Inc, Washington (1983).

Wig, N.N., Mangalwedhe, K., Bedi, H., Srinivasa Murthy, R. A follow-up study of hysteria. *Ind J Psychiatry* 24(2), 120–125 (1982).

Wig, N.N. and Parhee, R. *Classification of acute psychotic states*. Paper presented at WHO/ASEAN Forum on status of diagnosis and classification of mental disorders, alcohol and drug related problems in the Third World. Jakarta, Indonesia (1984).

Wig, N.N., Setyonegoro, K., Shen Yu Cun and Sell, H. Problems of psychiatric diagnosis and classification in the Third World. In *Mental disorders, alcohol and drug related problems: International perspective on their diagnosis and classification*. Excerpta Medica International Congress, Series 669, 50–60, Excerpta Medica Amsterdam (1985).

Wig, N.N. and Singh, G. A proposed classification of psychiatric disorders for use in India. *Ind J Psychiatry* 9, 158–171 (1967).

9
Sources and Traditions of Contemporary Spanish Psychiatry

Juan J. López-Ibor, Jr.*

Ancient Times

The history of Spanish psychiatry has been determined, just as any other aspect of Spanish history, by a constant interweaving of bonds that little by little have come to form a common nexus: that which is Spanish.

With respect to medicine in general and psychiatry in particular, the first one to be practiced with a scientific character was the Greek-Roman one. As such, it was brought to Spain in different periods. The most important author born in Spain was Lucio Anneo Seneca, although he spent all his life in Rome. His writings contain some interesting psychopathological ideas, for example, that inordinate anger produces madness or about the therapeutic use of the helleborus.

Lucio Vivio, who was very preoccupied with the so-called "furiosus," also acquired great fame. One of his inscriptions remains in the church of El Salvador in Seville.

Medicine leaned on humoral pathology and treatment methods derived from the late Alexandrian schools. Besides hysteria and epilepsy, great importance was given to the study of "melancholia" and its varied metamorphosis. A unitarian concept of the illness prevailed, without wanting to disperse it symptomatically, in order to differentiate it from healthy state. Isidoro de Sevilla (560–636), in his book *Las Etimologías* (600 A.D.), considered medicine as intimately interlaced with philosophy. This intimate union constituted the structure of the medical act.

For the time of Roman domination, the widespread use of the words "furiosus" or "amens" has to be interpreted as a predominance of the legal points of view. In a later stage the expressions "orates" and "endemoniados" ("bedeviled") took the lead and later still the word "inocentes" ("innocents," "those who are harmless") began to be used;

* Clínica López-Ibor, Madrid, Spain.

this considered them not responsible and as if in need of special protection and support.

If one wants to characterize in a few words what is peculiar to Spanish psychiatry (and to the understanding of human nature in general in this culture), I believe that one has to refer to the above-mentioned evolution of the concepts. First, a "Greek classical" perspective, bound to philosophical concepts, then a "Roman classical" legal perspective as contained in the words "amens" and "furiosus," overlaid later by Christian concepts (as in "endemoniados") which paved the way for a humanistic attitude in which those entrapped by madness are described as innocents. This linking of concepts is to be seen in almost any of the great transition periods of history, mainly in the 15th century, as well as nowadays.

But to get back to ancient times, Saint Cosme and Saint Damian distinguished themselves in the care of the insane in Seville. Both of them were tortured following orders from the Roman emperors Dioclecianus and Maximilianus in the year 303, but the devotion toward those saints persisted together with this new spirit that the innocents and mentally ill needed care and protection. Since then in Spain there exists what is called "Hermandades de San Cosme y San Damian" ("Brotherhoods of St. Cosme and St. Damian") made up fundamentally of physicians who want to give their clinical practice a religious sense and are dedicated in a special way to the care of the ill.

From the therapeutic point of view, the most important treatments were water cures in spas (Alange, Lora del Rio and many more, still in use today).

Middle Ages

The long period between the Arab invasion (711 A.D.) and the reconquest of the reign of Granada (1492 A.D.) was crucial to the formation of Spain. Not only because the Spanish language caught on, just as the historian Americo Castro has described, but also for the coexistence of the three monotheistic religions: Christian, Judaic and Mohammedan, an accomplishment of singular historic importance. There lies the true interweaving and one that shaped the characteristics of the Spanish people according to the great historian Sánchez Albornoz ("España, un Enigma Histórico"). Much earlier than in other countries in Europe, the Christians living in northern Spain started calling themselves by the modern natural term "Spanish," and many traces of art and history suggest that the Moors living in the south were also considered and considered themselves to be "Spanish."

The Arabs had places of seclusion for the insane from the 7th century approximately (Bagdag and Fez). In early times, between the 711 and 1200 A.D., the date of the founding of the first Spanish University at Palencia, scientific knowledge was in the hands of the moslems. Al-Hakem sent philosophers to Cordoba to translate the medical works of Hippocrates and Galen. But the classical tradition passed on above all through the Arabs by means of the so-called "Escuela de Traductores de Toledo" ("School of Translators of Toledo"), founded by King Alfonso the 10th, which contributed to the saving for posterity a good part of the cultural wealth of the epoch. Thanks to their work, many psychopathologic ideas of the classic age are conserved.

Psychiatry in "Al-Andalus"

For the Arabs, Al-Andalus was a province of a vast Empire comprising most of the present Spain, Morocco and neighboring countries. Since the Spanish Reconquest started in the North, the great division of Spain was established between Al-Andalus and the northern part of the peninsula. The distance between the Greco-Roman culture and that of the Arabs is enormous. The former is based on a human-centered world while the second is oriented toward the wish of Allah the Almighty. In architecture everything was built to draw attention toward what was *above* human height. Below this dimension lie only frail columns to support heavenly creations. The Greek culture, and the Roman even more so, were installed solidly on the ground from which everything stems upwards.

The extension of the Arab empire was supported by an interest in conquest, to which was closely linked another of the scientific type. Around the year 1000 Al-Bermin said that the sciences and knowledge of the whole world had been translated into Arab to achieve that new heart impelled by so many live currents that could start and sustain the new great organism formed.

The Greco-Latin heritage extended not only throughout the Christian West, but also throughout China, India, the ancient Orient, Byzantium and Africa besides all the area that formed Islam itself. The Arabs placed themselves between the Hellenic culture and the new Christian West and established a cultural diffusion greater than their conquests themselves.

The Arab doctor was a "hakim," that is, a medical philosopher, a sage. Thanks to language, there has not been any culture that has assimilated traditional learning better than the Arab. The individuals contributing most to psychopathological and psychological thought were the following (a very good summary of the legacy of the individual authors can be found in Ammar, 1965):

— Avicebrom or Ibn-Gebirol (1021–1071), who systematized Aristotles' knowledge about the soul. The vegetative soul produces the necessary movements for reproduction and growth, the vital soul for the sensations and movement, while the rational soul takes charge of thought.

— Avicena or Ibn-Sina (978–1036) was inspired by the teachings of Aristotle, although with some small variants in his doctrine. In his *Intelectus adquisitus* he describes human nature as being composed of body and soul. In the human soul a spiritual force is to be differentiated from a sensorial one. In his treatise *De anima* he describes the passage of the human spirit from potential intelligence to intelligence in action. In the spirit of man, besides a superhuman intelligence, there is an intelligent reason. In melancholia the brain is affected "per consensum," and the original cause could lie in the stomach, in the liver, in the spleen or in the uterus. Avicena described a case of "erotic melancholia": Once he was called to the country of Georgia in order to visit a nephew of its king. Avicena beckoned to the Chancellor of the palace and made him say the names of all the people in it while he took the pulse of the patient. Upon pronouncing the name of one of them, the pulse quickened, from which Avicena deducted that that was the person the patient had fallen in love with, assuring his cure if the person who inspired such love was given to him. In this sense Avicena described the pathogenic force of secrets, something rediscovered during the 19th century by Benedikt and incorporated in the psychoanalytical theories of Breuer and Freud. Ellenberger has delved into this aspect of psychological medicine in his *The Discovery of the Unconscious*. Avicena, of course, described an important psychophysiological reaction of this young noble gentleman and its application to diagnosis, not very much different from modern polygraphic examinations.

Avicena coincided on some points with Alfarabi and the sect the latter founded called the "Brothers of Purity"—though not completely because he did not consider matter as an emanated product, rather he shared with Aristotle the idea of a potential intelligence which converted into actual intelligence by experience, by the acquisition of knowledge and, on the other hand, by what God placed directly in it. Avicena knew that the brain had bilateral and symmetrical ventricles and distinguished which were the principal functions attributed to each of them. Although Galen and others assigned the physiological and pathological functions to the brain mass which filled by the "Neume," Avicena and Arabs in general thought that the brain functions were spread out in the ventricular system itself. For Avicena psychological alterations came about because of changes in the proportions of the composition of the encephalon, and he divided them into disorders of the imagination and those of memory or into another group, in which he included melancholia, mania, imbecility and dementia. For him black bile was the cause of fear and sadness, yellow bile of irritability and violence and the pituita of seriousness. The anomalies of the frontal brain produced disorders of perception; those of the middle brain, imbecility, and those of the fourth ventricle, disorders of memory. Avicena followed the description of Greek medicine of the symptoms of mania and melancholia as well as the description of the means for their treatment. In psychology he was a follower of Aristotle. Recently, Cruz Hernández has published an anthology of Avicena's metaphysics, relating it closely to Greek philosophy.

— Avenzoar (1072–1163), born in Peñaflor (Seville), was in general of more practical tendencies (he was an "experimentator").

— Abrilcasis (1106) had great inclinations toward surgery. "When melancholia," he says, "is produced by decomposed humidity and thick pituita you have to cauterize."

— Avempace (Ibn-Bajah), who died in 1163, occupies a special place among his contemporaries, since they were inclined toward the neoplatonic tradition. He thought that the soul had developed through the emanation of the "Nous." On the other hand, Avempace thought that, much as animals have instincts, so do human beings as well, and therefore the strength of the forces came from below until it reached the intellectual force, which was like an emanation of God.

— Averroes (1126–1198) let himself be influenced completely by Aristotle's ideas, and even when there were contradictions between the writings of Galen and those of Aristotle, he was inclined toward the latter. However, he did not conceive of the "Nous" in Aristotle's way because, following Alexander of Aphrodisios, he stated that the potential "Nous" was individual but not eternal since it disappeared with death. Furthermore, as Averroes was looking for an intermediate path between Alexander of Aphrodisios and Temistos, he stated that the potential "Nous" is not only a capacity whose need is shown by its activity, that it was at the same time active and with its own force, but that this "Nous" could not be individual as mentioned above, rather it was linked to the active "Nous" in which all persons participated. Each person only has the capacity of taking some active particles of this existential "Nous" in the same way that all persons have the capacity to see light. After death the "Nous" continues to exist but not individually, but rather as something common to all humans, and this is the "Nous" which human beings posses as an emanation from God. That is to say, in each individual soul there is a particle of the immortal spirit since it takes its origin in it. However, there are differences between individuals, according to whether the participation is major or minor.

Judaic Contributions

— Mosen Maimónides, who lived in Cordoba (1139–1205), represents the most outstanding of the Judaic tradition. The most interesting work of his from the psychological and psychopathological point of view is his treatise *Guía de descarriados* ("A guide to the lost ones"), a book that even now can be read and not only for its historical interest. His knowledge of psychopathology, according to Fidel Fernández, was not negligible for those times. "One should not consider demented," he said, "he who runs through the streets, throws stones or breaks household equipment, but also he who has his conscience blinded by one fixed idea, being normal in everything else that has no relation to this idea"—forming therefore the idea of "monomania." Because of his Jewish origin, he had to live a nomadic life, in spite of his great value.

— The most important work in Judaic scholastic doctrine was the book of Suhar. According to this author, God is shown by His word and in His activity and was, therefore, the creator of Adam Kadmon (Cadmo, according to Greek mythology). This original human is composed of ten forces from which are derived, on the one hand, the psychological or psychic faculties and, on the other, the virtues. A human being's spiritual and immortal soul ("Neschama") is one part of the spiritual world. The soul that supports life ("Ruach") belongs to the psychic world and respiration ("Nphesch") belongs to the third material world. Suhar was influenced by Plotino and Plato.

— According to the writings of Solomo ben Debuda ben Gabirol (1020–1070), all that is not God has matter and form, by which he mixed Aristotle's and neoplatonic doctrines with Judaic thought.

Other Contributions

— From Christian Spain it is possible to point out the forensic perspective of "Las Siete Partidas" ("The Seven Laws") by King Alfonso the 10th, the Wise, thus gathering the Roman tradition full of Christian humanitarianism, which for forensic considerations has had an enduring influence up to the present day. There the insane are considered "sicut infantes" ("as children") and therefore as irresponsible. From this epoch also emanates the distinction between "obsessio" and "posessio," a most important distinction reformulated by Jaspers' notions about the strangeness of delusional thought in comparison to the recognition that obsessive thoughts stem from oneself or, in other words, the distinction between "ego-dystonic" and "ego-syntonic" psychological experiences.

— Petrus Hispanus (1226–1277) was a Galenic doctor and a philosopher who followed the Aristotelian line. He dealt with astrology a great deal. His main book is the *Tratado de Anima* ("Treatise of Soul") discovered by Grabman in 1927 in codex 3314 of the Spanish National Library. He was Portuguese and exerted a great influence on the entire Peninsula.

— The personality of Arnaldo de Vilanova (1250–1313) was extraordinary. Although he probably was born in France, Diepgen is inclined to consider him Spanish because of the place where he carried out his activities. He was of Valencian descent (Peset, 1961; Ullersperger, 1954).

— Of Vilanova we know of the diversity of his inclinations and knowledge, given the epoch in which he lived. He was physician to some of the Aragon kings and as well an alchemist. In his *Practica Medica* ("Medical Practice"), he deals with mania and melancholia, attributing the former to a vice of the anterior cell of the head which at the same time deprives it of imagination, and melancholia to the animal spirit, which provokes fear, sadness and mutism. Wine is found among the foods that cause melancholia because upon burning the humors produces a black bile. Anxiety from excessive studying to the retention of menstrual flows or of rotten sperm is described also as the result of internal causes such as anger. It is worthwhile pointing out his small treatise on the interpretation of dreams in which he mentions the significance of dreaming for the different parts of the body. So, for instance, dreaming about one's underarms is equal to dreaming about one's own daughters, as they are always under one's protection, and to dream about the shoulders means dreaming of spouses because they are such a burden to man. He was condemned by the Inquisition because he tried to amalgamate Hippocratic principles with the veneration of devils.

— Raimundo Lulio was born in Mayorca in 1232 and died in 1272. He was Franciscan and a man of a reputation not very common for those times. Although he was not a physician, he dealt with medicine also. Carrera y Artan has devoted a very thorough study to the structure of the rational soul and of its forces in the writings of Raimundo

Lulio. According to his diagram, the combinations between the different activities of the soul could give rise to different normal or psychopathological characters. Normal activity of the soul demands or supposes the normal activity of all the principal faculties, which are: memory, comprehension and will; but if its functioning is not correct, the soul suffers a change in its activities, for example, a forgetful memory, an ignorant intelligence and a will directed toward hate more than toward love. He left the writing *Liber de instrumentu intellectus in medicina* ("Book on the instruments of the mind in medicine").

The First Psychiatric Hospitals

It can be argued that the first psychiatric hospital in the world was the one established in Valencia. It is true that the mentally ill were accepted in isolated rooms of earlier hospitals, and that they stayed with other patients when they were not so perturbing. In 1326, in Georges Hospital in Elbing, which belonged to the dominion of the Teutonic Knights, some cells were built in the so-called "Doll-haus." The same kind of cells are mentioned in documents of the City Hospital of Hamburg in 1375 and of the great hospital of Erfurt, reconstructed in 1385. In 1403, at St. Mary of Bethlehem Hospital in London, six male "mentecapti" ("deprived of reason") were housed. This also was the case in the Hôtel-Dieu in Paris, The Hospital of the Holy Trinity in Salisbury, in Bamberg, in Passau, in Regensburg, and so on.

However, a hospital dedicated solely and exclusively to the care of the mentally ill, separate from hospitals for the rest of the infirmed, did not exist prior to the one in Valencia. The most important facts in the history of Spanish psychiatry was the founding of the first mental asylum in Valencia in 1409. The story is the following: On February 24th of said year Fray Juan Gilaberto Jofre, monk of the "Orden de la Merced" was going to preach at the Cathedral in Valencia on the day of our Lady of the Forsaken when he saw a mob of youths insulting and throwing stones at a poor insane man. He shortened the sermon he had planned for the day's festivity and converted his preaching to an exhortation to found a hospital in which the different types of insane could be sheltered. When he finished his sermon and upon descending from the pulpit, waiting for him in the Cathedral entrance were several citizens from among the listeners, presided by Lorenzo Salom, who right then and there decided to contribute the necessary economic means to found a hospital to be called "Santa María de los Inocentes" ("St. Mary of the Innocents"). King Martin the 1st of Aragon granted the permit for its functioning and the consequent titles, and on February 26th of the following year Pope Benedict XIII granted the corresponding papal letter. It was inaugurated on the 1st of June of the year 1410 (Merenciano, 1950; Sempere, 1959).

The fundamental peculiarity of Father Jofre's initiative arises precisely from having seen a mentally ill person hounded and pursued by healthy persons in the alleys next to the Cathedral in Valencia. His purpose was to attend to them and try to cure them. It has been said also that Father Jofre, being a mercedarian, knew of the existence of establishments of this kind in the Moslem countries, but a thorough study of what these really were shows that they had the same characteristics that were subsequently presented by the "Hôpitaux Generaux" in France and other places in Europe. In Granada, during Moslem domination, there existed an edifice for the seclusion of asocial persons, the plans of which have been reconstructed. According to the facts collected by Delgado Roig, the construction of a hospital was initiated in Granada during the time of Mohamed V, construction beginning in the year 1356 and ending in 1367. It was situated in the suburb called Haxasir ("for Pleasure") and has always been called "house of the insane and the innocent." The description by Lamperez, the architect, says it was formed from a rectangular plan of two floors, and in its facade was placed a small portal with porticos on the four sides, each with a corridor. At the rear there was a patio with four staircases and four rooms at the corners. The porticos and galleries served as places for the taking of walks by the convalescing patients, and off the corridors the infirmaries were probably situated. Water came out of the mouths of lions, which today are placed opposite the "Torre de las Damas" ("Tower of the Ladies") in the Alhambra. In one of the rooms a series of buttresses left spaces in between, like small cells very similar to those constructed by Bar-el Moristan from Bagdad in the 13th century.

In 1425, King Alfonso V founded in Zaragossa a hospital called the "Virgen de la Gracia" ("Virgin of Grace") with an inscription on its facade which read: "Urbi et orbe" since any type of person could be admitted to it without distinction as to religion or nationality. In one of the pavilions of this hospital there existed a section for the mentally ill which caught fire and was rebuilt in 1829. This hospital gained fame because of its introduction of the so-called "moral treatment" of mental patients from the first moment of its foundation. By 1549 there were close to 100 mental patients committed to it.

The patients were in charge of cleaning the house, with the exception of the patients' rooms, and were as well in charge of transporting water, coal and firewood. They were engaged also in the pharmacy and in field work. In the same way, they carried in stretchers the ill and wounded who needed it, under the inspection of one of the keepers, whom they called "padre" ("father"). In 1859, Desmaissons also emphasized the organization of this hospital as well as the one in Toledo which seemed perfect for their time.

In Seville, in 1436, Marco Sancho (or Sánchez) founded the third insane asylum in Spain. It is told that he went around collecting the insane who wandered the streets. Many of the ill from nearby towns found refuge there, and some of them were sent to the spas to take the water cures. Henry IV, in 1481, took it under his protection; later the Monarchs Isabel and Ferdinand were protectors of this hospital. In 1456, another one was constructed in Palma of Mayorca.

One of the most famous psychiatric hospitals in Spain was the one called "Hospital de los Inocentes" ("Hospital of the Innocents") in the city of Toledo, founded in 1483 by the papal nuncio Francisco Ortiz, who put it under the patronage of the local church chapter. It was enlarged in the year 1700, using a spacious building called "Casa del Nuncio" ("House of the Nuncio"). The regulations inside were established in detail.

The one in Valladolid was founded in 1489 by Sancho Velázquez de Cuellar, auditor of the State Chancellory.

In Barcelona the general hospital, "Hospital de la Santa Cruz," was dedicated to all types of patients, without distinction as to nationality, that is to say, it was not a true psychiatric hospital. It was rebuilt in 1680. It seems that in the year 1412 they also brought in nuns and monks as well as disturbed people. Subsequently, in 1836, the Academy of Medicine put out a report proposing the construction of a new asylum and psychiatric hospital, and in that way another more modern hospital was erected following the advice of the most famous psychiatrist of that time in that city, Dr. Pi y Molist.

Bernardino Alvarez, founder of the first insane asylum in the New World, was born in Utrera in 1517 and emigrated to Mexico when he was 20. He took part with the militia in several acts of war, but later he alternated such activities with plundering gambling halls even if he had to do it with daggers. He was so violent that his companions came to name him the captain of the mob who were authors of evil conduct. They were arrested, but Bernardino Alvarez, taking advantage of the darkness of the night, jumped over the walls of the prison and escaped with three other companions who were less fortunate than he was since they were captured and died at the gallows. But Bernardino with better luck found refuge in the house of a woman from the district of Necaltitlan, who supplied him with weapons, a horse and money to facilitate his escape. In that way he was able to arrive in Acapulco from where he shipped off to Peru. There he gave up his former profession, became a business man and accumulated an enormous fortune. After leading such a hazardous life, upon his father's death, and when his mother told him the misfortunes that affected the family, Bernardino, regretting the depraved existence he had followed, surrendered to prayers, vigils and fasts, and took refuge in the "Marques del Valle Hospital" to give care and alms to the ill. There were so many that the hospitals of the colony could not attend to all of them. Upon returning to Mexico, he took special notice of the mentally ill, and, taking advantage of a house of Hernán Cortés, he conceived the idea of founding a new hospital for them. He requested a licence, acquired it and got down to work. In a short time he had inaugurated the first hospital for the mentally ill in the New World (1567).

Later on, Bernardino Alvarez decided to open another new center and, in 1568, opened a hospital at Oxtepec and then one at Xalapa in memory of the Viceroy by that name. He founded other hospitals in Havana, Guatemala, Antequera, etc. He encountered the collaboration of many people, up to the point of deciding to establish a religious order called St. Hipolito's. Bernardino Alvarez died in Mexico City on the 12th of August, 1584. Though he endured so many vicissitudes, very little remains of his work, least of all of the religious order he founded. Economic penury was extreme after the death of the founder, as can be confirmed by the different documents kept in the General Archives of the Indies in Seville. These documents also show the meticulousness and spirit of justice that characterized those Spanish-American foundations.

Modern Age

In 1492, after a dark autumn, it looked as though the new lights of the Renaissance were going to extend throughout Europe. In the years between 1590 and 1630, it seemed that finally the great Renaissance midday was going to take place. However, the historic reality indicates that irrationality flourished in the time of Bacon, Montaigne and Descartes. The assemblies of witches increased to such a degree that in the witches sabbath in Hendaya (a French city on the border of Spain), up to 12,000 of them gathered together. Witches proliferated in Catholic and Protestant countries. During the Enlightenment superstition had begun to be restrained, but "the madness" persisted as a "preternatural error" in the minds of many people. The Church and the Inquisition wanted to stop the confusion that existed between those possessed of the devil and the insane, a confusion frequent in the Middle Ages and in part in the Modern Age, to such an extent that Trevor-Roper recently assured us that Spain was the country where the *least* amount of witches were burned or punished, for the simple reason that they were considered to be ill, an opinion which Kamen expressed even more moderately (it is not irrelevant to this fact that the distinction already figures in The Seven Laws of Alfonso the Wise between "obsessio" and "possesio"). The inquisitor Alfonso de Frias stopped the persecution of witches in the second trial of the Inquisition celebrated in Spain, alleging their condition as mentally ill.

In that era admission to Spanish insane asylums occurred only when necessary, counting furthermore on the fact that as soon as the patients improved, they had a certain liberty, something which Cervantes gave testimony to, describing in El Quijote the episode of a patient who believed himself cured and was picked up by a messenger from the Archbishop.

In the following we review the more important authors and their contributions to psychiatric thought:

— Juan Luis Vives (1492–1540) was a humanist who enjoyed some fame in his own time. His psychological publications give him the right to appear in these pages. In this respect, we should underline views about the association of ideas. In his Tratado del alma ("Treatise on the soul") he leans, for such affirmations, not only on the external continuity of time and space, but also on the internal one, and states that the study of the human soul is indispensable to the educator, the priest, the politician, etc. The physician moves between body and soul, he adds. From this could be ascertained his continuous reference to the somatic part in order to reach the psychological level later. The mind should be healthy, and a person who does not have a healthy mind should be taken to the hospital in order to be cured. The perturbation of the imagination can produce disorders of mood. His detailed analysis of the passions has been meticulously expounded by Zilboorg, who has not hesitated to compare him to Freud.

— Andres Laguna (1499–1560) was called the Spanish Galen. He was born in Segovia and was Emperor Charles the 5th's physician. In his most well-known work, he dealt with the different opinions about the soul based on ancient Greek theories. He accepted Plato's distinction between the rational soul and the affective one, to which he added the natural soul or the vegetative one. With respect to dreams, he leans on Heraclitus' view as well as that of the Stoics, although he also refers to the opinion of Alcmeon when he assures us that sleep comes about because of the withdrawal of blood from the veins. Laguna represents the influence of ancient Greek medicine that reached the physicians of this era.

— Although not properly concerned with psychiatry but rather with psychology, one of the most famous writers of his time was Juan Huarte de San Juan (1530–1592). His book *Examen de ingenios para las ciencias* ("Examination of intelligence for the sciences"), published in Madrid in 1668, has been translated into many languages because of the fame it acquired. Following Plato's and Aristotles' influence, he mentions that the different dispositions of humans depend on three qualities: heat, humidity and dryness. He distinguishes between the vegetative, the sensitive and the rational soul. The three possess a kind of innate wisdom that determines the temperament of each one. If at a certain moment humans succumb to an illness such as a mania, melancholia or frenzy, it is because the temperament of their brain has changed—and the reverse can occur if they are cured. He cites several clinical cases in favor of these affirmations, for example, the one of a frenzied woman who threw up in the face of whoever visited her his virtues or worse still, his vices, because "warmth is next to the orient of the spirit." Climate and cultural environment exercise an influence on the spirit. With increasing culture, mental illnesses increase. Climate has an influence over passions ("influences of subtleties") says Huarte. He also discussed in several publications the education of children, physiognomy—where Pujasol followed him— and the diversity of the mixture of racial influences constituting Spanish temperament. Finally, he assumed that the brain was the site of mental illness centuries before Gall, Esquirol or Griesinger.

— Luis Mercado (1520–1606) was the royal physician of Philip II and Philip III. His main work is divided into three parts. In the third one he deals with melancholia, repeating ideas of the Ancient Greeks. In the second he deals with a number of disorders such as epilepsy, frenitis, lethargy, melancholia and hypochondria.

— Francisco Vallés (or de Covarrubias) (1524–1592) discusses in his book *Sacra Philosophia* whether demoniacal illnesses exist and require the same therapy as those of other causes. He concludes that they do not exist, and that melancholia and epilepsy are produced by natural causes. Vallés finds it very important to separate exorcisms, predictions and prophecies of the Bible from the auguries and magic of the Romans and Arabs, i.e., to separate the mental illnesses—for him amentia, dementia, mania, insane furor and melancholia—from disorders that should not be considered illnesses, but rather vices, such as lust, irascibility and avarice (which reminds us of the distinctions between psychoses and variations of the psychological way of being of Kurt Schneider). Melancholia is not produced without the appearance of the melancholic humor or fluid extended in the brain itself if the influence is adequate, or in another part if it is by "consensus."

— An important author in the restoration of Greek medicine in Spain
  was Cristophoros de Vega, physician to the Infante don Carlos (son
  of Philip II) and professor of medicine at the University of Alcalá de
  Henares in or about the middle of the 16th century. It is known that
  he died in 1573. In his works he deals with manias, which he considered synonymous with insanity and rage. He also dedicated an
  extensive chapter to melancholia, relating its genesis to the plethora
  of blood and of black bile and to grief, sadness and troubles. He
  wrote about "flatulent melancholia," later dedicating special chapters to lycanthropy and erotomania. In order to treat the latter, he
  mixed medical measures with moral advice, such as distractions,
  games, reunions, excursions to pleasant places, and so on.

It is curious to point out that this Hellenic tradition of the origin of
melancholia should coexist with another from the Moslem tradition, so
that, for example, the royal physician of Charles the 5th, Luys Lovera
de Avila (1540), in his work *Quiebra en el regimiento de la salud y en la
esterilidad de los hombres y mujeres* ("Collapse in the management of
health and in the sterility of men and women"), leans totally on Avicena and assures that when the after-birth fluids were cut from mothers
these contracted melancholia, and he also cites as an origin of this
illness the termination of menstruation.

— If only briefly, one must mention Oliva Sabuco de Nantes, although
  according to some, the author of the book was really her father.
  Other authors have said that some notable Arab or Jewish physician
  who escaped from persecution in Alcaraz must have been the person
  who initiated Doña Oliva in the study of philosophy and medicine.
  She wrote a dialogue on the *Naturaleza del hombre* ("The nature of
  man") and another on *Vera medicina* ("True medicine") (1587). Her
  knowledge of psychology may be considered very superior to her
  psychopathologic knowledge, and thus she studied the different
  emotions and sentimental states knowing the heart and human cus-
  toms very well.
  To the brain, she says, come all the sensations of all the injuries and
  external damages of the body, and it is because the body is the
  beginning and cause of the feeling. In another section she states that
  Spaniards follow the common custom of wearing black without any
  reason or motive since that color saddens as does light and darkness.
  Her thinking shows some peculiarities that remind us of Heraclitus,
  for example, when she writes that maturity and perfection denote the
  beginning of imperfection and decay, that health is the cause of
  illness, and where there is life there is death. Life is a tedious death
  always decreasing and taking away life. The principal and general
  remedy of the *Vera medicina* is to form the soul in Purgatory with the

body and remove dissension, and the best remedy consists of words which, in adults, engender joy and hope for the best. From these statements she developed a treatise on psychotherapy.

— Andrés Velázquez published a book about melancholia in 1585, a book with a Galenic spirit. In the fifth chapter, he explains the meanings of the word and the mechanisms of its origin. However, he completes the study referring to how, besides the known symptomatology, in some there appear qualms of conscience, in others prodigality, whereas still others feel like a cock trying to cluck and beat its wings and others feel like a brick and do not dare drink anything for fear of dissolving, etc. He maintained the unity of mania and melancholia.

— Gómez Pereira wrote the famous *Antoniana Margarita* (Valladolid, 1605) in which he contradicted the Galenic points of view. "Animals do not have a sensorial life, rather they let their organs be influenced by objects or phantoms." He rejected the idea of animals having sensitive souls. It is not known whether this rejection was spontaneous or guided by his religious sentiments.

— Alfonso Ponce de Santa Cruz, physician to Philip the 2nd, wrote a book about melancholia published in 1622—one of the most interesting in the history of Spanish psychiatry. It is divided into several dialogues about the nature and origin of melancholia, its symptoms and treatment. The melancholic humor is a product of bile which attacks the brain. When this humor affects the memory, it produces sadness, fear and anxiety. If the point of attack is the womb, uterine furor is produced, and if the humor attacks hypochondriacs and is accompanied by obstructions, then it engenders hypochondria. In this casuistry there are curious observations such as that of the patient who believed he was converted into a glass and covered with straw for some time until he was cured, remitting his delusion and stating that no such monomania existed, but that he was really an unfortunate man (this is the theme of the *Licenciado Vidriera* by Cervantes). Another 30-year-old patient succumbed first to sadness, then to monomania, which even transformed him into a wolf (lycanthropy), making him flee from men and take refuge in the mountains where he spent the nights howling as well as visiting cemeteries and calling to the dead.

— The former should not be confused with Antonio Ponce de Santa Cruz, his son, royal first physician to Philip IV, who died in 1650.

— Esteban Pujasol wrote *Anatomía de ingenios* ("Anatomy of intellect") (1637). Previous authors had divided the brain into three spaces. In the first and frontal one lay common sense, fantasy and imaginative force; in the second or middle one lay the intellectual force and judgment; and in the third lay memory or the faculty to remember. From the physiognomical point of view he wrote, for example, that a large head denotes virtue and sagacity, bravery and strength in his inner senses, and that whoever possessed such is prudent and wise. He put forth other commentaries like the above relating the size and form of the head with the characteristic features of the patient. The third part of his work is a type of treatise on astrology dealing with the influence of the stars on temperament.

— Francisco Nuñez de Oria in his *Regimiento y aviso de sanidad* ("Management and notice of health") (Madrid, 1562 and 1572), deals with the influence of food on good habits. A sanguine nature brings with it good understanding and straight judgment. The melancholic one is sensitive, sagacious and docile. The stoic is a normative and cold. And the angry one is daring, sudden and sharp.

— Tomas Murillo Velarde y Jurado was born in Belalcazar and was physician to King Philip IV and to Charles II. His work was entitled *Aprobación de ingenios y curación de hipocondriacos* ("Endorsement of the ingenious and curing of hypochondriacs") (Zaragossa, 1672) in which very particular observations and remedies are referred. The work does not contain anything original, apart from maintaining that witches and devils can really engender melancholia, and that the Devil has his seat in the spleen and the black bile. He considered hypochondriacal melancholia to be produced in the entire body, although one is bound more to the brain.

— Andres Piquer (1711–1772) was one of the great medical celebrities from Spain, physician to Kings Ferdinand VI and Charles III. In his treatise he describes convulsions, tremors, epilepsy, vertigo, frenitis, insomnia, lethargy, catalepsy, coma, apoplexy and paralysis, melancholia and hypochondriac affection. In another of his manuscripts he deals especially with the final illness of the King, most probably of Ferdinand VI, according to Chinchilla, the well-known historian of Spanish Medicine. Piquer writes:

Although his Majesty seemed to be well during the time of the illness the Queen died from, he was repugnant already to carry out life's everyday things such as eating, sleeping and going to the countryside. The temperament of the King is melancholic and is inclined to this state by his own nature so that even being healthy he has some fears that are only found in those possessed of melancholia; and the illness that his Majesty already suffered years ago, which lasted thirteen months, shows us amply that this Prince has melancholic blood in abundance. The ailment began to manifest itself with very vivid fears where he feared dying or suffocating or that he would suffer an accident. Together with this he did some things which seemed extravagant, attributed to geniality, although I thought they were occasioned by the illness. Because a few days hence he started to leave the handling of his affairs, he left his hunting, he did not allow the cutting of his hair or his beard and in this way other little things which clearly indicated his ailment. He slept well but every time he woke up the fears and melancholia were greater than before and because of this he left his bed and placed himself in a little miserable bed, which is the one he keeps today. He believed also that the meals exasperated him because after them he felt more worked up by the melancholias (. . .). He suffered great fears, believing that he would die at any moment, because he felt he was suffocating, because he was being destroyed inside or because he was going to have an accident. This he said and repeated so many times and with such vehemence, that they were innumerable (. . .). He adhered to and was fixed to these sad and melancholic ideas, without giving occasion to talk about other things (. . .). His Majesty had the fixed idea since five months ago of death being accompanied by a great anxiety, in such a way that when I was with him he had no other conversation.

— It is very difficult to find in modern literature a more accurate though short description of major depression. This manuscript is reproduced in Volume IV of the *Historic Annals of General Medicine of Spain*. Piquer insists that mania and melancholia are one and the same illness, distinguished only by the grade of morbose activity of the spirit.

— Gaspar Casal became established as a physician in Oviedo after having been one in Madrid. He wrote a work entitled *Historia natural y médica del Principado de Asturias* ("Natural and medical history of the Asturias Principality") (Madrid, 1762), published after his death by Juan Carlos García Sevillano. He took care of the endemic in that Principality and describes mania or furious insanity as endemic to the town of Piñola. In another chapter he speaks of the frequency with which epilepsy is associated with melancholia; but his principal merit lies in having described the psychological symptoms of what was then called "sickness of the rose" (pellagra).

Contemporary Age

The last years of the 18th century are testimony to great social transformations which culminated in the French Revolution and which did not leave psychiatry out. The transformations in care (Tuke, Pinel) represented the indispensable preamble to the surge of scientific psychopathology (Esquirol). Psychiatric hospitalization in Spain had been maintained within limits of quality and humanitarianism superior to the rest of Europe. Pinel himself, traveling with a young Scottish psychiatrist (most probably with William Cullen himself) admired the organization and care of the "Hospital de Gracia" in Zaragossa and later incorporated its philosophy and methods into his moral treatment which was at the core of the scientific and psychotherapeutic approach to psychiatry founded by him and his disciple Esquirol. However, the hardships of the 19th century had negative consequences on our psychiatry. The alienation of all church properties, including mental hospitals, by the laws of Mendizabal ended up in the little that still remained, and the 19th century ended with a much worse system of care than had developed in the greater part of Europe and North America—and, more importantly, worse than what existed here 100 years previously.

Ignacio María Ruiz de Luzimiaga (1763–1822) and Ramón López Matías deserve to be mentioned. The former wrote a dissertation about manias and another about a treatment for dementia, nourishing both dissertations with the experience he had acquired in England. Ramón López Matías in 1810 wrote a book about the "demons or those possessed of the devil" half in fun and half seriously. In another work published in 1810 he discussed the problems of disturbance of reason through external causes, insisting on the power of melancholia, especially the religious one, and of the persistent mania, setting forth the problem from the forensic perspective. His fundamental preoccupation was that of determining the freedom with which humans act in those cases and the relationship between the offence and the punishment. From the philosophical point of view, besides Descartes, Kant, Fichte and Schelling, Krause had a great influence on López Matías.

The great influence of French psychiatry on Spanish psychiatry started in the 19th century through Pinel and Esquirol, although one should not forget that Cullen in his time was already translated and read by Spanish physicians. The most well-known men of the era were Pi i Polist, Pedro Mata (1811–1877), José María Esquerdo (1842–1912), Jaime Vera (1859–1918), Juan Giné i Partagas (1836–1911) and Arturo Galcerán Granés (born in 1850). Pedro Mata took up the most important point for the defence of insanity which is the differential diagnosis between crime and insanity. It should be stated here that the problem of the defense of insanity is considered very differently in countries of northern Europe from those of the south where Roman law has had a significant influence. Defense of insanity in England has always been biased by actual facts, namely an impressive series of attempted or assumed magnicides which culminated in the MacNaughton case. Daniel MacNaughton, probably a schizophrenic, surely responding to his delusions of a persecutory nature, was acquitted for reason of madness but the subsequent social response led to the formulation of the MacNaughton Rules by the House of Lords, rules according to which Daniel MacNaughton would probably have been executed.

In the Spanish forensic tradition, since "The Seven Laws" of Alphonse the 10th, the crucial question was not whether insanity is present or not, but the way it affects the act of the offence itself, leading to the need for a psychopathological analysis of the criminal act and the distinction between those relating to insanity and those that are not. There is an interesting in-between state, one of a normal psychological state of abnormal intensity, but one that remains in the realm of normality. Pedro Mata set a set of rules to differentiate the "act of reason" from the "act of madness or insanity," among them that the latter lacked an "internal history" which permits psychological differentiation of the one from the other. From a psychopathological point of view, his notion was very similar to later ones of Jaspers when he distinguished between "process" and "development."

A. Pujadas (1811–1888) founded the psychiatric hospital of San Baudillo de Llobregat in Barcelona, and he tried, without success, to develop a scientific psychiatry. He published within two years the *Revista de Medicina e Higiene Mental*, the first Spanish scientific journal devoted to psychiatry and mental health. Financial problems of the hospital were great until, after Pujadas' suicide, the Order of San Juan de Dios (1895) took charge of it, entrusting its direction to Galcerán, who later was the director of the "Pedro Mata Hospital" in Reus (Tarragona). He collaborated in the *Revista Frenopática Española* (founded in 1881) and in *Archivos de Terapéutica de Enfermedades Nerviosas y Mentales* (1904). In Madrid in 1886, Esquerdo founded the sanatorium that bears his name.

In the 19th century scientific decadence was accentuated. Marañon, a great physician of the present century, in a work about half a century of psychiatry, when referring to the 19th century mentions only a few names: José María Esquerdo, Jaime Vera, Perez Valdés (1853–1927), Nicolas Achúcarro (1880–1918) and Sanchis Banús (1890–1932). Two different groups extended into the 20th century. For some of them, such as Esquerdo and Jaime Vera, in spite of their great talent and gifts as practical psychiatrists, politics attracted them more than science. Different reasons sterilized the work of R. Pérez Valdés and R. Valle Aldabalde (1863–1937). Achúcarro was more inclined toward pathology.

The appearance of Ramón y Cajal seemed to free a decadent Spain from its inferiority complex. His work and models resulted decisively in the creation of a new atmosphere in experimental science. Ramón y Cajal was a histologist and his most well-known discoveries were on the histology of the nervous system. In their connection as more or less close disciples of his, the following stand out: Tello, Villaverde, Lafora, Prados Such, Castro, Río-Ortega and a few others. But actually, Cajal's preferences as a researcher did not include psychiatry. It is interesting to quote the following text of his:

I have to allude to Freud and criticize some of his most audacious observations. Because in more than five hundred personal dreams that I have had analyzed (without counting the ones of persons I know) it is impossible to prove, except in very rare cases, the doctrines of the bold and somewhat self-worshipping Viennese author, who has always seemed to me more preoccupied with the idea of establishing a sensational theory than with the wish to austerely serve the cause of scientific truths.

Also, as Kraepelin mentions, Ramón y Cajal was never well acquainted with the developments of psychiatry in Europe.

In the bosom of this "cajalian" stage of Spanish medicine, immersed in the spirit of "'98"* and with the urge to make a base for a scientific Spanish psychiatry, emerged a new generation of psychiatrists, many of them trained in Austria, Germany, England, the United States, Switzerland and other countries, grouped in two large urban centers of the country. In Barcelona (Figure 1), Pi i Molist, Giné i Partagás and Mira López stand out. In Madrid (Figure 2) besides Pedro Mata, José María Esquerdo and Jaime Vera, who have already been mentioned, Luis Simarro (1851–1921), Conrado Rodríguez Lafora (1886–1971), J. Sanchis Banús, José María Villaverde, (1888-1936), José Miguel Sacristán (1889–1957) and Antonio Vallejo-Nágera (1888–1960) are prominent. Sanchis Banús was the promoter of the concepts of "enajenación" ("insanity") and "trastorno mental transitorio" ("transitory mental disturbance") collected in the Penal Code for the insanity defense (in the law which reflected involuntary admissions to psychiatric institutions which prevailed from 1931 to 1984).

Also from this time are the present-day psychiatric journals: *Archivos de Neurobiología* (1920), *Actas de Psiquiatría y Neurología* (1940, today called *Actas Luso-españolas de Neurología, Psiquiatría y Ciencias Afines*), *Revista de Psicología General y Aplicada, Revista de Psiquiatría y Psicología Médica de Europa y América Latina* (1952), and scientific psychiatric societies: Liga de Higiene Mental, Asociación Española de Neuropsiquiatría, Sociedad Española de Psiquiatría, Sociedad Española de Psiquiatría Biológica, etc.

During the last years of the Second Republic (1931–1936) and the first ones after the Civil War, the first Chairs in Psychiatry were established at Spanish universities; until then psychiatry had been taught in the Faculties of Medicine as a part of Legal Medicine. E. Mira López was granted a Chair in Barcelona (although he did not appear in the National roster as it was not a national Chair, but one created by the Catalan Government). Others included Antonio Vallejo-Nágera, Ramón Sarró and Juan J. López Ibor (who has held the Chair of Legal

---

* The 1898 generation of intellectuals and writers encompasses authors embroiled with the melancholies of the loss of the Spanish Empire, the impoverishment of Spain, and the loss of meaning of the Spanish culture, arrogant in face of the French Revolution, forgetting its enlightened past, which lost not only an empire, but a sense of identity as well in a long process that ended, so we would like to believe, with the end of the last century.

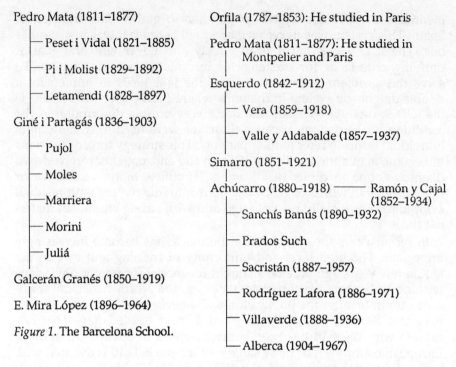

Figure 1. The Barcelona School.

Figure 2. The Madrid School.

Medicine, Toxicology and Psychiatry since 1932). Román Alberca and Luis Rojas Ballesteros were the first psychiatrists to accede to the highest post of a teaching career. With that, Spanish psychiatry reached its coming of age.

Spanish Psychiatry Today

Although the French influence was most important in the last century, Kraepelin has had a deep influence on Spanish psychiatry in this century. Up to the Spanish Civil War and World War II, the German influence was overwhelming, and the classifications used were German (i.e., Reichardt's). After the Civil War several chairs and training centers in psychiatry were implemented. Most of the Heads of new departments had had at least part of their training in Germany, though everyone tended to develop his own classification system.

In the 1950s the PANAP ("Patronato Nacional de Asistencia Psiquiátrica"), the branch of government responsible for psychiatry, implemented a classification system of its own to gather data from all of Spain. This system was never well accepted because it was just another one. The ICD 9 was never used widely and never with the goal of unifying criteria or for exchange of information among centers. To solve this problem, I have tried since the late 1960s to implement a double diagnostic system in the units where I have been active. One is the ICD 9, the other a "personal one," very often a description of the condition of the patient, because clinicians were used to coining quite individual terms to refer to their patients. This strategy forced clinicians to become acquainted with the ICD. In the end patients received two diagnoses, one in digits (ICD) and a lengthier, more descriptive or dynamic one in words (e.g., 295.2; "schizophrenic patient with residual symptoms, not socially rehabilitated and with strong emotional maternal links.")

In recent years the Anglo-Saxon influence has become increasingly important. The high level and uniformity of training and care in the U.K. a few years ago became a sought-for model for young physicians wishing to become psychiatrists. Later on, the North American influence caught on after the publication of *Comprehensive Psychiatry* (Freedman and Kaplan) and DSM-III filled a most needed gap. That can explain why DSM-III has been better accepted in Spain than in other European countries. For these same reasons the ICD 10 is awaited with hopeful expectations.

There are no official classification requests on the part of the central authorities in Spain. Psychiatric clinics and hospitals have to report to the Ministry of Health according to the PANAP or similar classifications. No such requests are made in general hospitals nor in community medicine, and the Social Security System (which finances the bulk of the health care in Spain) seems to be uninterested in diagnoses. With the transformation of Spain into the present federated country, health care is in the process of being transferred to local governments ("Comunidades Autónomas"), each one with different criteria and approaches.

Three principal authors of the post-Civil War period can be mentioned: Sarró, López-Ibor and Llopis. Sarró, trained as a psychoanalyst and endowed with a rich clinical and philosophical knowledge, became interested in a topic outside the core of early psychoanalytical writings: delusions, and has been able to describe the main topics of all delusions, which are limited in number and coincide with the topics of myths described the anthropological sciences ("mitologemas"). Schizophrenic delusion represents a powerful creative impulse to control a reality where meaning is no longer possible and opens the windows to a reality beyond reality which, by being so suprahuman, is in fact so very human.

López-Ibor, on the other hand, found his attention drawn toward neurotic and psychosomatic disorders and, well aware of the limits of psychoanalytic theory, was able to discover some unexplainable facts in them. In other words, neurotic anxiety could not be fully explained through biographical childhood family events, but had an endogenous element within it. Neurotic anxiety was analogous to endogenous sadness ("vital sadness" according to K. Schneider) and therefore called "vital anxiety." López Ibor proposed the term "timopatía ansiosa" for these endogenous disorders different from the neuroses, but later he said that the cause of every neurotic disorder was this vital anxiety. Furthermore, vital anxiety was to be treated with biological methods: Fiamberti's acethylcholine shocks in the early 1950s, MAOI and tricyclic antidepressants later on. DSM-III and the studies of Klein and Sheehan have brought to our attention these descriptions of López Ibor's made in the late 1940s and the 1950s based on sound clinical examinations of patients and on a solid philosophical background able to analyze the undescribed psychobiological foundations of psychoanalysis. For López Ibor, Freud's anthropological notions are directly connected to the traditions of the gnostics (López Ibor, 1972).

A third contribution should be mentioned. The experience of the occurrence of the mental disorders related to pellagra after our Civil War led Bartolomé Llopis to call attention to the old notion of "the single psychosis," a theory embraced by Griesinger and very recently by Janzarik himself. In this case, a single ethiological factor, pellagra, is able to produce the whole realm of psychopathology, from neurasthenic manifestations to dementia, including depressive, delusional and confusional disorders.

Final Remarks

Science has no boundaries, and the problems of applying scientific knowledge to the solutions of practical problems, i.e., the care of patients, seem nowadays to be the same all over the world. Nevertheless, the history of certain countries is responsible for some peculiarities in the personality of psychiatry in different parts of the world and constitutes a treasury of reflections. Insanity, psychological disturbances and the definition and care of those affected by them always raise the same problems, which come time and again to the forefront of discussion by psychiatrists. Huarte de San Juan, Voltaire, Esquirol, Griesinger, Wernicke and many others defined madness as mental illness and mental illness as brain disorder, to be almost immediately questioned by their contemporaries embracing psychological or social points of view. The struggle between "somaticists" and "psychologicists" in Germany early in the 19th century, or between psychiatry and anti-psychiatry all over the world in the last two decades, is neverending.

In any case, it is worthwhile to reconsider the past of our traditions in order to delve into the approaches they have used to face such perennial problems. From the detailed mention of the history of psychopathology in Spain a few points can be summarized:

First, of course, I have always referred to the term psychopathology and not psychiatry because psychiatry as a medical specialty was not born as an independent discipline until the first decades of the 19th century. But psychopathological knowledge was consistent with medical knowledge much more then than now.

Spanish medieval medicine was embodied with deep philosophical aspects that even transcended religious beliefs, in a piece of land where Christians, Moslems and Jews found a place in which to live together and in which to fight each other. Arab and Christian kings and landlords never hesitated to look for the best physician available, no matter what their religion. A physician had to be a sage, a hakim, learned in philosophy and human knowledge. Modern Spanish psychiatry is still endowed with philosophical and anthropological values. For instance, the same year that Breuer's and Freud's initial paper on psychoanalysis was published, 1892, two translations appeared in Spanish, one in Barcelona and another in Granada (Carles Egea). From then on psychoanalysis became quite accepted in intellectual circles, although perhaps not in psychiatry so much. The first translation of Freud's complete works was the Spanish one—a beautiful one to be sure. On the other hand, the influence of modern post-Hegelian philosophy on Spanish psychiatry, either directly or through Spanish philosophers (Ortega y Gasset, Unamuno, D'Ors, Zubiri and others), is very important but generally without losing ground or clinical experience, something which makes this approach still modern.

A very significant trend of Spanish psychiatry is in forensic psychiatry. The "Siete Partidas" ("Seven Laws") of Alfonso X settled the rules that for centuries have been applied to the judging of the insane. The early distinction of the Spanish Inquisition that witchcraft had nothing to do with heresy, but that it was related more to medicine (something referred to later on by Weyer in what Zilboorg called the "first psychiatric revolution") also helped in this sense. This approach has two main characteristics: one is humanitarian and Christian, the other one psychopathological. Pedro Mata, as he mentioned a century ago, described the rules to distinguish acts of reason from acts of madness. The essential aspect here is the psychological analysis of the offence itself in order to judge whether it originated by madness or not. The clinical diagnosis of the offender or his symptoms are secondary to the problem itself. It is the *act* that must be analyzed. Among the rules, several refer to what years later Jaspers described as the comprehension and explanation of symptoms or to the "Sinngesetzlichkeit" of K. Schneider's psychopathology. In the early 1930s these aspects shaped a new Penal Code to which the category "enajenación" ("insanity") and "trastorno mental transitorio" ("transient mental disturbance") was incorporated, which was very important in the evaluation of offenses in epileptic or toxic conditions. The problem in the defense of insanity is more straightforward, humanitarian and scientific than in the English-speaking countries, where a series of attempted magnicides from George IV to Ronald Reagan have confused the problem.

In the last decades biological psychiatry has had a deep influence on Spanish psychiatry, paving the way for new nosological approaches such as DSM-III, which, interestingly enough, has gained a great deal of acceptance in Spain.

The trend toward unification of psychiatrists, tendencies is a potent one nowadays. It has originated in psychiatry itself. The training of a psychiatrist in Spain is controlled by a National Commission (a "board") with highly unified programs, and many psychiatric units in the university system and general hospitals have become aware of the importance of unifying criteria, standardizing methods and exchanging clinical information among themselves and beyond Spanish borders. That is to say, the generalization of a common instrument for diagnosis (such as ICD 10) in Spain will depend more on the attitudes of psychiatrists than on those of the Health Authorities, and it will have a primary impact on training, research and the care of patients—depending, of course, on the quality of the instrument used and on the political aspects of same (DSM is a national system, "too North American"; ICD is international).

But psychiatric care, hurt by the laws of Mendizabal of the early 19th century and never fully recovered afterwards, is suffering from the impact of anti-psychiatric perspectives, trying to be enforced in an epoch of political transition from an autocratic to a democratic political system. Nevertheless, the development of scientific psychiatry all over the world is the only way to promote better systems of care.

References

Only basic and general texts are provided, as many of the original contibutions are difficult to find in ordinary libraries.

Ammar, Sleïm: *En souvenir de la medecine arabe. Quelques uns de ses grands noms.* Bascone et Muscat. Tunis, 1965.

Cervantes de Salazar, F.: *Life in the Imperial and Loyal city of Mexico in New Spain and the Royal and Pontifical University of Mexico as described in the "Dialogues" for the study of the Latin language (1554).* University of Texas Press, Shepard, Austin, Texas, 1953.

Chamberlain, A.S.: Early Mental Hospitals in Spain. *Amer. J. Psychiat.*, 123, 143–149, 1966.

Chinchilla, A.: *Anales históricos de la medicina en general y datos biográfico-bibliográficos de la española en particular.* López y Compañía, Valencia, 1841.

Delgado Roig, J.: *Fundaciones psiquiátricas en Sevilla y el Nuevo Mundo.* Paz Montalvo, Madrid, 1948.

Desmaisson: L'assistance aux alienes chez les arabes du VIII au XII siecle. *Ann. Med. Psychol.*, 96, 689–709, 1938.

Dieckhöfer, K.: *El desarrollo de la psiquiatría en España. Elementos hitóricos y culturales.* Gredos, Madrid, 1984.

Ellenberger, Henri F.: *The Discovery of the Unconscious.* Basic Books, New York, 1970.

Ferrer Hombravella, J.: Aportaciones a la historia de la psiquiatría española. *Medicina Clínica*, 11, 440–451, 1948.

Foucault, M.: *Historia de la locura. Breviarios del Fondo de Cultura Económica.* México, Madrid, Buenos Aires, 1976.

Howells, J.G.: *World History of Psychiatry.* Brunner/Mazel, New York, 1975.

Kamen, H.: *The Spanish Inquisition.* G. Weidenfeld and Nicholson, London, 1965.

Kraepelin, E. *Lebenserinnungen.* Springer, Berlin, 1986.

López Ibor, J.J.: *Freud y sus ocultos dioses.* Editorial Planeta, Barcelona, 1972.

López Ibor, J.J. & López-Ibor, Jr., J.J.: Historia de la Psiquiatría Española. In: *Psiquiatría, Vol. I.* Eds: C. Ruiz Ogara, D. Barcia Salorio & J.J. López-Ibor, Jr. Toray, Barcelona, 1982.

Mata, Pedro: *Tratado de la razón humana.* C. Bailly-Bailliere, Madrid, 1878

Merenciano, F.M.: Vida y obra del Padre Jofre. *Arch. Ibero-amer. Hist. Med.*, 2, 305–359, 1950.

Mora, G.: From Demonology to Narrenturm. In: *Historic Derivations of Modern Psychiatry.* Ed: I. Galdson. McGraw-Hill Book Company, Montreal, 1967.

Peset Llorca, V.: Una introducción a la historia de la psiquiatría en España. *Med. Clin.*, 369–379, 1961.

Sánchez Albornoz, C.: *España, un enigma histórico.* Buenos Aires, 1957.

Sarró, Ramón: La historia franco-alemana del delirio, desde Pinel a Binswanger. In: *Psiquiatría, Vol. II.* Eds: J.J. López-Ibor, Jr., D. Barcia Salorio & C. Ruiz Ogara. pp. 868–894. Toray, Barcelona, 1982.

Sauri, J.J.: *Historia de las ideas psiquiátricas.* C. Lohlé. Buenos Aires, Mexico, 1969.

Sempere Corbi, J.: *Como nació, como era, como funcionaba el "Hospitals dells folls de Sancta Maria dels Ignocents."* Real Academia de Medicina, Valencia, 1959.

Ullesperger, J.B.: *La historia de la psicología y de la psiquiatría en España.* Editorial Alhambra. Madrid, 1954.

Watt, W.M. & Cachia, P.: *History of Islamic Spain.* Edinburgh Univ. Press, Edinburgh, 1965.

Zilboorg, G.: *A History of Medical Psychology.* W.W. Norton, New York, 1941.

Subject Index

Person Index